Stephanie Oakes'
Burn Off 10 Pounds
a Month

The Ultimate Exercise Program
for Quick (and Lasting) Weight Loss

Stephanie Oakes

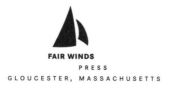

FAIR WINDS
PRESS
GLOUCESTER, MASSACHUSETTS

First published in the USA in 2006 by
Fair Winds Press, a member of
Quayside Publishing Group
33 Commercial Street
Gloucester, MA 01930

10 09 08 07 06   1 2 3 4 5

ISBN 1-59233-160-2

Library of Congress Cataloging-in-Publication Data

Oakes, Stephanie.
  Stephanie Oakes' burn Off 10 Pounds a month / Stephanie Oakes.
      p. cm.
  Summary: "Workout programs using walking as the source of exercise"—
Provided by publisher.
  Includes bibliographical references.
  ISBN 1-59233-160-2
  1. Walking. 2. Fitness walking. I. Title: Walk off 10 pounds a month. II.
Title: Walk off ten pounds a month. III. Title.
  GV502.O18 2006
  613.7'17--dc22   2005024250

Cover design by Howard Grossman/12E Design
Book design by *tabula rasa* graphic design
Photography by Allan Penn

Printed and bound in USA

The information in this book is for educational purposes only. It is not intended to replace the advice of a physician or medical practitioner. Please see your health care provider before beginning any new health program.

This book is dedicated to my two boys, Lucas and Nicholas.

Contents

Acknowledgments

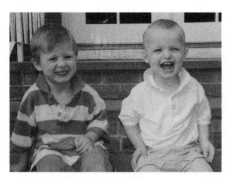

After 20 years in the health and fitness industry and numerous television appearances and articles, people routinely asked me "when are you going to write a book"? Well I suppose it took two children to get me off the circuit for a few months so that I could dedicate the time and effort required for such an intensive undertaking. However, never could such an undertaking be achieved alone and there are several people who believed in me and helped contribute towards the successful completion of *Burn Off 10 Pounds a Month,* for which I am deeply indebted. First, to those for whom I wrote this book, there is a way to achieve effective results in losing weight through walking, and I encourage you to participate and thank you for your insights solicited during the research for this book. Thanks also to my very good friend Michael Yardis for his valuable research and creative workout programs. They are a terrific blend of varied, creative yet effective techniques.

I'm grateful for my parents, Phil and Julie Oakes, who taught all their children and grandchildren that preventative medicine is the best kind and to always enjoy some form of movement, activity, and/or sport. Thanks to Beth Henry, who encourages me to "always write."

Michael Maxtone-Graham, your many articles, anecdotes, creative advice, and encouragement are so very appreciated.

Chris thanks for helping to keep our lives active, creative, and fun.

Introduction

Walking for a Slimmer You

I HAVE WORKED IN THE HEALTH AND FITNESS FIELD for more than 20 years and I have been exposed to just about every form of exercise equipment, new fad, and diet imaginable. Yet I have found that *nothing* is as enjoyable or as effective for weight-loss as taking long, frequent walks. Perhaps because it is one of the simplest forms of exercise, taking a walk is also one of the most underestimated. It seems I'm not alone. *Time* magazine conducted a poll for their June 6, 2005, cover story titled "Lose that Spare Tire" asking Americans their preference for exercise routines. Sixty-nine percent said they walk for exercise (more than any other activity). My husband (and walking partner), Chris Graham, refers to walking as "driving slow with the top down, except you're the vehicle!" You can take time to enjoy the view, commune with nature, and even ponder deep thoughts. Yet don't be fooled: Walking can be a terrific workout.

Walking is one of the great common denominators in life. It is the one form of exercise that virtually everyone can do, whether you're in your twenties or your seventies, whether you have 10 pounds to lose or 50 (or more). I've often wondered why more of us haven't discovered the secret of incorporating a walking regime into our daily lives, but unfortunately we've become more a nation of sitters instead of walkers. The demands of the office, the lure of 500 TV channels, or the responsibilities of our families have erected barriers to obtaining what is our natural birthright—a healthy, lean, strong body.

Government statistics make it very clear that today, millions of Americans are becoming rounder and rounder. Added pounds have an insidious way of suddenly appearing, and before you know it, your trim waistline is history. And while most of us realize that carrying extra pounds can lead to dangerous, often life-threatening, health conditions—including heart disease, diabetes, and stroke—many of us feel overwhelmed when it comes to choosing (and then following) an exercise plan that will help us shed those unwanted pounds. For many, going to the gym every day is either not practical or simply not a way we want to spend our precious time. Fortunately, you don't have to become a gym rat or invest in thousands of dollars of expensive exercise equipment to get fit, melt pounds from your body, and feel stronger and more energized than you have in years. Instead, all you need to do is start putting one foot in front of the other. I know, because it worked for me. When I was 5 months pregnant with my second son, Nicholas, and carrying around my 7-month-old, Luke, many unsolicited comments came my way: "Don't worry, dear, you'll lose that weight one day."

Believe me, after having two back-to-back pregnancies and C-sections (my boys are 16 months apart), I found that my waistline was staunchly resisting going back to its former state. Many acquaintances even suggested a tummy tuck, but that's just not my style. Still, my scale kept insisting that I weighed much more than I wanted to...and where was all my muscle tone?

Now, before you think I'm whining a bit too much, consider that I've spent my entire working life in the health and fitness business, and it's always been my policy when it comes to a physical training program not to demand more of my clients than I demand of myself. Don't get me wrong, I've certainly had other setbacks, including a scuba-diving injury that took me out of the game and put me in rehab for 12 months. After that injury, it was walking that slowly brought me back to good health. Now, faced with post-pregnancy weight and feeling less than happy with my body, I decided that I had to do something—quickly, before I started experiencing all the negative effects of poor health.

After a lot of research and planning, I decided that my best bet for weight loss would be my old friend: walking. And so I designed a walking plan that I was determined to follow religiously. I felt that any plan I developed should include these six critical elements.

1. The routines must fit easily into my often-hectic schedule.

2. They must be healthy, with no risk of injury.

3. They must keep me stimulated and never bore me.

4. They must not require a lot of expensive equipment.

5. They must build muscle tone.

6. And finally, they must enable me to lose up to 10 pounds each month.

Now I don't have to tell you that a walking plan that could meet all these requirements would definitely *not* be like any of the plodding routines our mothers used to undertake from time to time. This was to be a scientifically designed program that would get me back in shape again.

Today I'm thrilled to tell you that it worked like magic. I'm now back to my former weight, and my pre-pregnancy clothes all fit perfectly again. As you might expect, a lot of my friends were curious to know how I'd accomplished this "miracle" (no surgeries, thank you!). And, of course, I was delighted to pass along my secret to them and my clients.

I was also thrilled when I was invited to share my walking program with a wider audience by writing a book that describes all my walking routines in detail, making it easy for anyone who wants to lose weight to follow them. These are unique "boot camp" routines that I designed especially for busy people who are interested in a fast and effective weight-loss program.

Because you're now holding this book in your hands, I imagine that you are one of these interested people. And so I want to welcome you to a brand-new world of walking that I am convinced will make you a thinner *and* a happier person.

More than 2,500 years ago, the Chinese philosopher Lao-tzu proclaimed: "A journey of a thousand miles must begin with a single step." I invite you to turn the page and join me on that momentous first step.

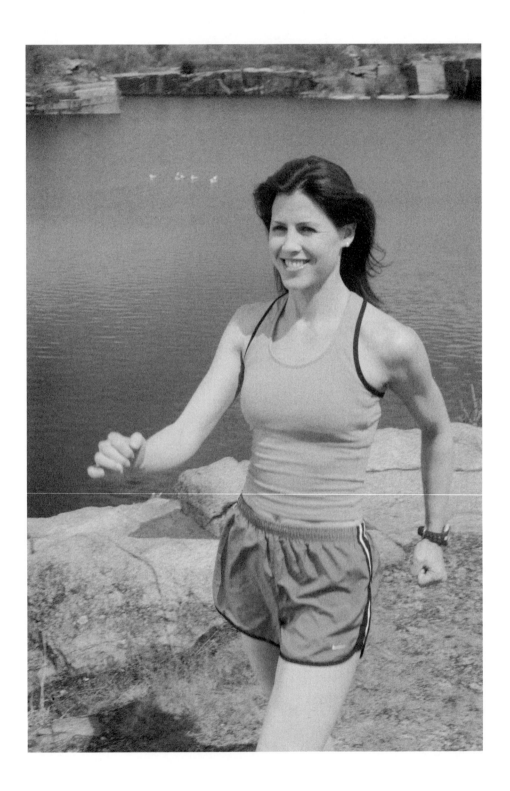

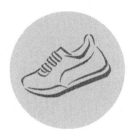

PART ONE

Walk Off
the Weight

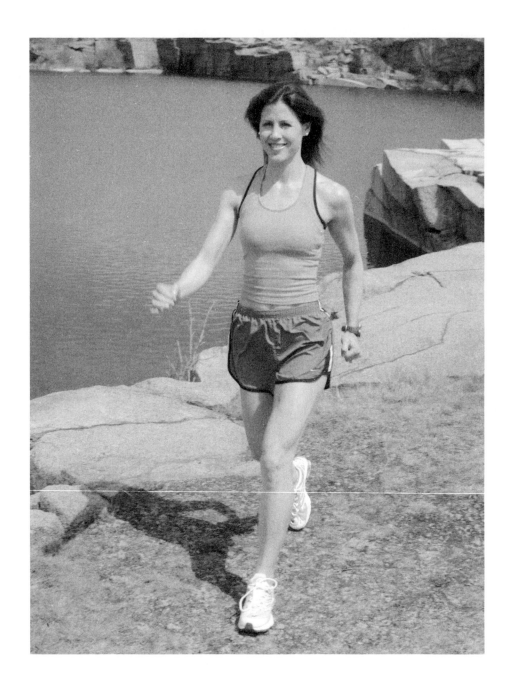

"Walking is man's best medicine."
—Hippocrates

CHAPTER ONE

Walking: Still the Perfect Exercise for Weight Loss

I T HAPPENS TO THE BEST OF US. One day, we notice we have to fasten our belts one notch looser than we had before. Clothes that once were comfortable are now snug. Elastic becomes our friend. We notice that simple things we do every day, like carrying a bag of groceries, climbing a flight of stairs, or hoisting our kids or grandkids onto our laps, suddenly seem a lot harder. We're out of breath more even when we do less.

The reasons for gaining weight are as diverse as the readers who pick up this book. Perhaps you suffered an injury or illness that kept you off your feet for a number of weeks. Calories you used to burn throughout the course of the day instead started to add up, packing on the pounds. Maybe your doctor prescribed medication that, as a nasty side effect, caused your body to gain weight more easily, even though you didn't increase the number of calories you consume. Perhaps you gave birth recently (or not so recently), and you've had trouble losing those pregnancy pounds. Or maybe you ate your way through a stressful event—a job loss, the illness or death of a loved one, or a move to a new city where you knew no one—and now, though your life has started to run a bit more smoothly, you find yourself carrying a lot more pounds than you used to.

For most of us, though, the reason for our weight gain isn't anything quite so dramatic. For the majority of people, weight gain goes hand in hand with this frantic, breakneck-pace life we all lead. Many of us start to feel as though our cars are our second homes as we rush to work, to school, to appointments and meetings and soccer practice and, finally, back home. By the end of the day, we're so exhausted that it's a struggle to get a meal on the table, much less think about *exercising!*

So despite our best intentions, we end up eating a diet that is full of sugar, caffeine, and processed foods and getting little to no regular exercise. We promise ourselves that tomorrow, or this weekend, or next month, we'll start eating better, working out, and paying more attention to our health. But tomorrow never seems to come, does it?

In the end, though, *how* you gained the weight doesn't really matter. It's what you plan to do about it that counts. And because you've picked up this book on walking, you've already taken (yes, pun intended) the first step. Unlike the thousands of people who complain that they've gained weight but haven't yet done anything about it, you, my friend, are on your way. For whatever reason—an upcoming class reunion, the simple desire to look and feel better, the urging of your doctor—you are now ready to *do something* about your weight gain. And the good news is that you're just a workout away from making progress.

For Weight Loss, Simplicity Equals Success

In this world of high-speed digital Internet access, instant messaging, and satellite-monitored onboard navigation systems in our cars, the idea of *simplicity* seems as dated as, well, putting a stamp on a letter and dropping it in a mailbox. So when it comes time to pick an exercise method to lose those unwanted pounds, it may seem only natural to think high-tech. And if that's what you're looking for, there are plenty of options available—just take a tour of your local gym. But consider this: As an effective weight-loss method *that can be maintained long term,* nothing beats walking.

Not convinced? Consider this simple fact of human biology: In order to lose weight, the number of calories you expend during the course of the day must be greater than the number of calories you take in. That's it! And exercise is, of course, the best way to increase your calorie expenditure for the day.

Think of it this way: Your body's metabolism is much like the engine in your car. If you leave your car parked, but running, it will eventually run out of fuel. But if you drive it around all day, accelerating, going up and down hills and across town, you're going to have an empty tank much sooner.

Now, here's the important thing: After your body uses up the "fuel," or calories, you fed it today, it then begins to burn the fuel stored in your body already. Guess where it goes first? Fat cells. So if, for example, you consume 1,500 calories a day, but your body needs a total of 2,000 calories per day to get you through your daily activities plus your walking workouts, then you've created a 500-calorie deficit for that day. Over the course of a week of this same regimen, you will create a 3,500-calorie deficit, which equals 1 pound of fat. Gone, off your body. Do that every week this year, and you will lose 52 pounds.

The math seems pretty simple. So why, then, is taking off the pounds so darn hard? When people are unsuccessful in their efforts to lose weight, it's usually not because they didn't burn calories with whatever exercise method they chose. It's most often because their exercise plans got derailed. A lack of time, lack of commitment to get to the gym, simple boredom, or injury resulted in their giving up. To lose weight, you've got to consistently burn more calories than you take in. In other words, you've got to keep at it, and I'm convinced that the easiest weight-loss strategy *to keep at* is walking.

Now while it's true that, compared to walking, some other types of exercise will burn more calories in a shorter amount of time, most of these are high-impact activities. And as a result, they have substantially higher rates of injury. What's more, when you're injured, it's hard—and often unsafe—to continue working out. And needing to take frequent breaks to recover can sap your motivation as well as your momentum. So we've come full circle. In the end, walking wins out because it consistently burns calories *over the long term.*

Think of all the reasons you've had in the past for giving up—or not starting— an exercise routine: The gym didn't have convenient hours, or perhaps you felt self-conscious there with all those studly guys and abs-baring women. Maybe you could never find the time to fit in a workout. Or you got bored with the routine. Perhaps you tried your best, but you got hurt, and it was hard to get back in the swing of things after being laid up for a couple of weeks.

Walking is the perfect antidote to all of these exercise busters. In fact, it may just be the world's most perfect exercise. Here's why.

Efficient calorie burn: Think about this pair of statistics for a moment.

• For every mile we walk on level terrain, we burn approximately 100 calories.

• For every mile we *run* on level terrain, we burn approximately 100 calories.

Now, who wants to pound the pavement? Raise your hand, please. Hmmm... I didn't think so. The truth is, a program of regular walking will burn off unwanted pounds safely and effectively—and keep them off. To lose weight, you don't have to run a marathon. All you need to do is consistently burn more calories per day than you take in, and walking will help you do that.

Low risk of injury: I'm willing to bet that you know a few former runners who got sidelined because of injury. Maybe you even fit into this category. And when you consider the physics of running, it's not hard to see why injuries are so common: With each step, running places forces of *6 to 12 times* your weight on your body. Doing the math, that means that the average person is absorbing forces of 900 to 1,800 pounds with every step they take running. On the other hand, when you walk, your body absorbs forces only equal to your weight, which means that you're a lot less likely to get injured. And because you're much less likely to get injured, you're much *more* likely to maintain your fitness program for the long haul.

All This, And Weight Loss, Too!

Although your main goal in starting a walking program may be to lose weight, you'll also be doing your body a huge favor in other ways. Here are 10 invaluable health benefits you'll gain when you follow my structured walking program.

1. A stronger cardiovascular system. In fact, regular walking can decrease your resting pulse rate, which means your heart doesn't have to work quite so hard to get you through the day.

2. A reduced risk for a heart attack. Based on his landmark study of 17,000 Harvard alumni, Dr. Ralph S. Paffenbarger, Jr., concluded that a daily 2-mile walk can reduce the risk of a heart attack by 28 percent or more. Walking lowers levels of low-density lipoprotein (LDL) cholesterol (the "bad" kind) and raises levels of high-density lipoprotein (HDL) cholesterol (the "good" kind). A regular walking program also reduces your risk of developing high blood pressure, a factor that contributes to heart disease and stroke. And if you already have high blood pressure, walking can help reduce it.

3. A stronger immune system, which increases your odds of fighting off infection and disease.

4. Increased bone density, which lowers your risk of developing osteoporosis.

5. Increased circulation to your joints, which can result in less pain for people with arthritic joints.

6. A reduced risk for developing type 2 diabetes. And if you already have the disease, taking part in a regular walking program can improve your body's ability to process sugar (known as glucose tolerance), lower your blood sugar levels, and help you live longer.

7. Increased mobility and stamina.

8. Improved posture, resulting in fewer backaches.

9. Stress relief and greater mental functioning. Going for a brisk walk is a great way to reduce stress. Regular walking also can reduce feelings of depression and anxiety.

10. Improved ability to stay strong and active through the years. Walking for physical fitness can improve your balance, which becomes even more important as you get older. A regular walking program can help you prevent falls, keep you mobile, and help you maintain your independence.

24/7 convenience: As a busy mother of two young boys, I sometimes find myself fitting in exercise at strange hours—late in the evening, early in the morning, whenever my youngest takes a nap. If, like me, you sometimes wonder when you're going to find the time to exercise given everything else that needs to be done during the day, then walking is the answer. No need to depend on the local gym's schedule or to get yourself to a class at a predetermined—but oh-so-inconvenient—hour. When you're walking for weight loss, you can work out whenever is most convenient for you. Simply lace up your shoes and head out the door. And if you can't find the time for an extended walk of, say, 30 minutes straight, you're the perfect candidate for my Now and Later program, which allows you to get in your daily exercise requirement in short bursts of as little as 10 minutes. (I'll explain it in detail on page 103.)

What's more, if your career or lifestyle takes you away from home for long periods of time, you don't need to halt your walking routine (unlike most other fitness programs). If you find yourself in a new city or with time to kill in an airport, you can still get in your walking workout. (I'll explain the Business and Vacation Travel workout on page 111.) Again, consistently working out over the long term means weight-loss success.

No previous experience needed: When it comes to weight-loss methods, walking is the equal opportunity employer of the fitness world. Whether you have fond memories of being a sports star in high school or your memories are more likely to center on getting picked last in gym class, *you can succeed* at the walking programs in this book. My detailed instructions and targeted plans make weight loss a no-brainer. As long as you're willing to commit to the plan, you *cannot* fail. What's more, once you start shedding pounds through these routines and begin to experience how good it feels to be fit, you're likely to embrace the inner athlete that resides in all of us.

Note: While walking is typically safe for everyone, be aware that because the walking programs in this book are designed for fast, effective weight loss, they will be challenging for some people. If you have been sedentary lately or have a pre-existing medical condition, such as an increased risk for heart disease or stroke, be sure to get your doctor's okay before beginning any exercise program, including the walking routines in this book. For additional precautions, see "Before You Walk, Have a Talk" on page 35.

Minimal expense. In chapter 3, I'll list the walking "equipment" you'll want to invest in before starting out. But, fortunately, the list is pretty short, with the main items being a good pair of properly fitting walking or running shoes (if you're of a certain age, you probably know them better as "sneakers"); some synthetic or merino wool socks; and an inexpensive, no-frills pedometer. If you plan to walk at night, you'll also want to get some inexpensive reflective tape to place on your shoes. (Safety first, always!)

Along the way, you might also choose to get yourself some snazzy exercise clothes that will add to your comfort (and give you style points) as you work out. But they are entirely optional, and doing my workouts doesn't mean you need to break the bank buying a new wardrobe. In fact, walking is probably the least expensive workout option available.

The Fun Factor

Okay, so walking is a top choice for weight loss, it has a low risk of injury, it can be done anywhere, at any time, and it costs next to nothing. But are you worried that it's going to be *borrrring?* Fear not.

The programs in this book have been specially designed to keep you interested and motivated. Unlike walking programs in other books, you won't be doing the same workout day after day. Instead, you'll be mixing it up. In the course of a week, you may complete five or six different walking workouts—taking you everywhere from around your neighborhood to the mall to a treadmill and beyond—and a variety of specially chosen stretches and strength-training moves. There are three good reasons why I've designed my program this way.

1. First and foremost, mixing up your workouts is the best way to achieve overall fitness. Why? Because by doing so, you're constantly throwing new challenges at your muscles, forcing them to adapt and get stronger with each workout.

2. Mixing up your workouts keeps you interested and motivated, allowing you to look forward to a new challenge every day.

3. Having workout options helps you fit your exercise program around your schedule—not the other way around. So if, for example, it's raining, you can choose to do the Mall and Museum Walks or hop on a treadmill. Busy taking care of your baby or grandchild? Try out the Baby, Stroller, and You workout program, which will help you burn calories while keeping your child entertained. (I'll explain the programs in detail in chapter 5.)

Welcome to a New Era in Walking Workouts

Is it really possible to lose up to 10 pounds a month with my walking routines? Go ahead and flip to part two of this book (page 53) and check out the workouts there. I think you'll quickly realize that *these are not your mama's walking routines.* There will be no strolling through a park. No ambling down the block, hand in hand with your partner, gazing at the sunset. To borrow a phrase from celebrity chef Emeril Lagasse, "We're going to kick it up a notch."

I've designed the revolutionary workouts in this book for fast, effective weight loss. In order to lose up to 10 pounds in a month, you're going to be taking walking to a whole new level. Sure, you'll still be putting one foot in front of the other, but each step will be part of an overall, custom-designed plan to lose a targeted range of calories each and every week, with a total weight-loss goal of up to 10 pounds in a month. Think of it as boot camp for the walker. (In chapter 2, I'll explain in precise detail how to use the programs in this book.)

Though challenging, these workouts are based on solid science. In 2005, federal health officials issued new, tougher exercise standards as part of their dietary guidelines. Like the old guidelines, the new ones recommend at least 30 minutes of moderate activity on most days of the week. This figure translates to walking 2 miles in 30 minutes, or the equivalent. The new guidelines also say it may take an additional 30 minutes a day, for a total of 60 minutes, to prevent weight gain. Finally, they call for another 30 minutes—90 in all—to sustain weight loss in previously overweight or obese people.

The program in this book is designed to meet these new guidelines for weight loss and maintenance. The exact amount of weight you will lose depends on a number of factors, including your current weight, metabolism, gender, and age. However, if you do your best to follow the program, you are virtually guaranteed safe, effective weight loss.

Boosting Your Fitness with Strength Training

In addition to my walking workouts, you'll also be completing my targeted Strength-Training Workout two or three times each week. These exercises will help you build lean muscle mass. The duo of burning calories through walking and gaining lean muscle through strength-training moves is bad news for those unwanted pounds wearing out their welcome on your hips, thighs, and belly. Why? Muscle is calorie hungry. One pound of lean muscle mass requires 35 calories every day just to maintain itself. On the other hand, 1 pound of fat tissue requires only 2 to 3 calories per day. This is the magic pathway to weight loss: Add lean muscle mass that requires calories and then tap into the stores of fat on your body for this additional energy need. The result? Lost body weight, in the form of fat tissue.

This is why every successful weight-loss program requires three components: aerobic exercise such as walking that efficiently and effectively burns calories;

strength-training work to build lean, calorie-hungry muscle; and, finally, a healthy eating plan. We've already got the first two components covered with the workouts in this book; now let's briefly discuss the third.

Eating for Weight Loss

We all know that eating a healthy balance of nutritious foods is a central point to weight loss and maintaining a healthy weight. Recently, the U.S. Department of Health and Human Services confirmed that almost two-thirds of Americans are overweight or obese. One reason is because more than half get too little physical activity or eat too much junk food.

There are myriad diets out there, and I'm not here to tell you which one is right for you. I strongly recommend that you discuss your diet options with your doctor or a dietitian. If you have certain medical needs—such as a history of heart disease or diabetes—your eating plan will need to be custom-tailored to address these concerns. Here, however, are a few general guidelines for healthy eating.

Think long term. Your friend may have lost an incredible 50 pounds on a cabbage broth diet, but that doesn't mean that her weight loss is healthy. Avoid any diet that requires you to eat only one food or type of food. You want a diet that you can sustain over the long term, not a fad. Whatever diet you choose, it should allow you to eat a variety of foods, in balanced amounts. The diet that is right for you depends on your medical history, the types of food you prefer (and those that make you feel the best), and your lifestyle.

Consider if five meals a day is right for you. Many nutrition experts and athletes believe that eating five smaller meals throughout the day is better than eating three big ones because a steady food intake keeps your energy levels higher. Plus, you'll be less likely to feel starved before a meal, which means you'll be less likely to overindulge. The trick is choosing the right foods and controlling the portion sizes. For more on proper portion size, see "Is Your Portion Size Affecting Your Waist Size?" on page 24.

Be snack smart. One of the easiest things you can do to improve your diet is to replace fat-filled snacks such as potato chips and ice cream with healthy ones. After all, food is your body's fuel, and just as putting a high-octane gasoline in your car keeps the motor humming, putting "high-octane" food in your tummy keeps your body running smoothly. So choose your snacks carefully. For a sweet treat, make a smoothie by throwing some fresh fruit, low-fat yogurt, and crushed ice in your blender and giving it a whirl. Or opt for an ounce or so of low-fat cheese and a few whole grain crackers. Following are a few other ideas for healthy snack foods that will fuel your body and help you get all the nutrition you need.

Apples: At 100 calories for a medium apple, the fiber, carbs, and vitamins provide a great snack.

Bananas: A great source of potassium, bananas also contain vitamin B6. A medium-size banana has about 105 calories.

Carrots: For crunch and a touch of sweetness, reach for carrots, which are a great source of beta-carotene and vitamin A. A medium-size carrot has 30 to 40 calories. For the ultimate in convenience, buy bags of peeled baby carrots and reach for them whenever you want a quick snack.

Whole-grain cereal with fat-free or soy milk: Most cereals are fortified with vitamins and minerals, and they're great with fresh fruit. Individual-size boxes of cereal have between 200 and 400 calories with milk or soy milk added. Just be sure to choose a low-sugar, high-fiber cereal.

Low-fat fruit or soy yogurt: A top source of calcium, yogurt also contains protein and potassium. All that for just 250 calories per 8 ounces!

Nuts: My kids love the protein-packed tamari almonds. Ten to fifteen nuts contain 150 calories.

Reduced-fat peanut butter on whole-grain bread: This tasty snack is high in protein as well as fiber and other minerals.

Choose the food that took the shortest trip to your plate. The more a food is processed, the more likely it is to contain hidden fats, sugars, and preservatives. Whenever possible, choose food in its natural state, like fresh organic fruits and veggies, fresh rather than prepackaged meats, and fish like salmon, trout, and albacore tuna. Olive oil, almonds, walnuts, soy, whole-grain breads, brown rice, and fresh beans are terrific choices as well. These foods actually go beyond basic nutrition and help fight disease to make us healthier.

Don't skip breakfast. The cereal commercials are correct: Breakfast really is the most important meal of the day. After you go a long period without eating (such as overnight), your blood sugar levels will be low. Skipping breakfast can mean your body will start to crave something sweet, and you'll end up snacking on unhealthy foods. Also, if you go too long without food, your body thinks it's starving and will begin to store fat. So it's best to begin your day with a nutritious meal to jump-start your metabolism.

Stay hydrated. Unless you've been living in a cave, I'm sure you've heard the dictum to "Drink eight to ten 8-ounce glasses of water a day." But did you ever wonder what was so magical about that particular amount of water? During the course of a day, even one in which we don't "work out," our bodies lose a huge amount of water simply in the process of keeping us alive.

We lose water through respiration—in other words, each time we take a

Is Your Portion Size Affecting Your Waist Size?

I'm always amazed that in restaurants (fast food and otherwise) I can fill up by eating off the children's menu, which offers portions half the size of the adult portions. In recent years, portion sizes have grown, well...out of proportion. As consumers, we may think we're getting good value for our money, but the truth is that large portion sizes can have a direct impact on our waist sizes. So keep the following portion sizes in mind when you prepare your meals or order in a restaurant. (If the restaurant offers only one size of the item you're ordering, simply divide the food into the proper portion as soon as you get it and immediately ask for a doggie bag.)

- One serving of vegetables or fruit = size of a baseball
- $\frac{1}{2}$ cup of cooked rice or pasta = a rounded handful
- A serving of meat, fish, or poultry = the palm of your hand (don't count your fingers!) or a deck of cards
- $\frac{1}{4}$ cup of dried fruit or nuts = size of a golf ball
- $\frac{1}{2}$ cup of ice cream = size of a tennis ball
- One serving of pancakes = size of a compact disc
- One teaspoon of peanut butter = size of your thumb tip
- One serving of cheese = size of six dice

For more information on portion sizes, take a look at the recently published USDA Food Guide Pyramid at www.nal.usda.gov/fnic/Fpyr/pyramid.html.

breath. We lose it in the form of perspiration, or sweat, and even when we aren't aware that we're sweating, water is still evaporating off our skin, through our body's built-in temperature regulation process. And, of course, we lose water when we urinate. Just how much do we lose? Though the exact amount varies depending on the individual and factors such as the temperature and humidity of our surroundings, the average is about 2½ quarts every day—or approximately 80 ounces! So it turns out that the advice to drink 64 to 80 ounces of water a day isn't at all arbitrary. This amount of water simply replaces the amount of water we've lost through normal processes. Add in exercise, and you're running in the red, water-wise.

What's more, we often mistake thirst for hunger. This means that what we may think is a craving for a snack might just as easily be satisfied with a glass of ice water (and a lot fewer calories).

Fill up on fiber. Just because you're trying to lose weight doesn't mean you need to feel hungry all the time. Foods that are high in fiber tend to make you feel fuller, longer. So be sure to eat plenty of beans, fruits, and vegetables. And unless you're on a low-carb diet, take advantage of the appetite-suppressing benefits of whole-grain cereals and whole-wheat breads. As an added bonus, these foods are all nutrient-rich, so you get a bigger bang for your buck, nutrition-wise.

Limit your alcohol consumption. The average alcoholic beverage contains between 100 and 150 calories. That's why having a few drinks a week can slowly pack on the pounds. Plus, alcohol is a diuretic, which means it dehydrates you. And the first place we begin losing water is in our muscles. Weakening our muscles will make our workouts even more difficult, making it harder to exercise efficiently and lose weight. For all these reasons, keep your intake of alcoholic beverages to no more than one per day.

For further advice on healthful diets and choosing the eating plan that's right for you, see my list of suggested books in "Recommended Reading" on page 175.

Taking the First Step

You are about to embark on a wonderful journey—a journey to a new, slimmer you. As you shed pounds, you'll be gaining energy and the newfound confidence that comes from meeting your goals. This journey will also be a journey of discovery, as you get back in touch with your body, perhaps feeling muscles you haven't felt in ages. You'll probably be surprised by your body's amazing ability to grow stronger as it becomes leaner.

You'll also discover things you hadn't noticed before about the world around you. We miss so much when we zip through our neighborhoods locked inside our cars. By hitting the pavement (or, better yet, getting off-road), you'll discover sights, sounds, and smells you had missed: the sight of a butterfly perched precariously atop a flower, just before it flutters off on a breeze, the smell of a freshly mowed lawn in the summertime, the sound of kids playing in the park. It all awaits you, and it all starts with a single step.

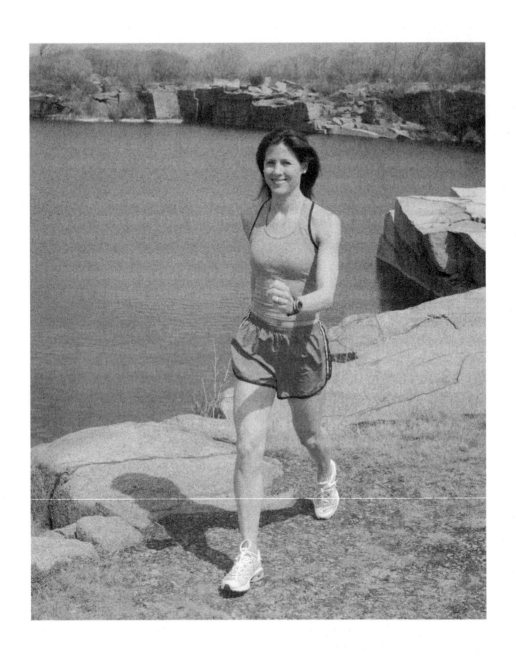

*"Walking is the best possible exercise.
Habituate yourself to walk very far."*
—Thomas Jefferson

CHAPTER TWO

How to Use This Book

ONCE YOU GET STARTED on one of my walking programs, the momentum you create will keep you moving and motivated. (After all, what better motivation is there than seeing your waist, thighs, and butt getting smaller!) But I'm well aware that *starting* an exercise program is often the hardest part. Many exercise programs fall into one of two categories: Either they require you to follow a rigid workout schedule that allows for absolutely no deviations from the plan (completing ignoring the fact that life doesn't happen on a set schedule), or they give you some broad brushstrokes of what to do but leave it up to you to figure out how best to construct a plan that is safe and effective—something that most people find overwhelming. Obviously, neither of these options is practical. That's why the workout program I've created is different. In my program, you'll get the best of both worlds—without any of the drawbacks.

The exercise program in this book gives you flexibility to choose from a number of workout options each day—giving you the freedom to make allowances based on the weather, your schedule, or simply your mood. Yet no matter which option you choose, you'll have the confidence of knowing that the workout you're doing is part of an overall custom-designed plan for safe, fast, effective weight loss. I've taken out the guesswork, but left in the flexibility. In this chapter, I'll explain in detail exactly what you'll be doing over the next weeks and months, so there will be no surprises. And in chapter 3, I'll detail the few pieces of gear you'll need. To learn how you're going to shed pounds, firm up, and feel better in just 1 month—and then repeat that feat month after month—read on!

Walking Workouts 101

My exercise program is built on 16 unique walking workouts, all of which can be found in part two of this book. Why so many? First, variety helps to keep you interested. I would never ask one of my clients to complete the same workout day after day, and I won't ask you to do that either. Second, each workout challenges your body's muscles in a slightly different way. Science shows that the best way to get strong is to constantly create new challenges for your body. When you do, your body is forced to constantly adapt—which, in biological terms, means get stronger. And finally, giving you a variety of workouts to choose from each day allows you to pick the workout that best suits you in that particular moment. So, for example, if it happens to be raining that day, you can choose to do the Treadmill Walking workout or my special Mall and Museum Walks workout. If, on the other hand, day care is closed and you need to combine child care with getting a workout, you can do my fun but challenging Baby, Stroller, and You workout. Woke up feeling a little stiff? Try out my No Joint Pain Necessary workout. Planning a round of golf this weekend? Check out my Walking for the Fairway workout. I think you get the picture.

Now while a major component of my program is flexibility, I'll still be guiding you every step of the way, making sure you're getting a well-rounded, safe, and effective workout program. To see what I mean, please turn to page 57. Consider these calendars the "master plan" to your exercise program. As you can see, each day when a walking workout is scheduled, I give you two or three options to choose from. Yet no matter which option you choose, I've specially arranged the workouts so that by the end of the week, you've gotten a complete, calorie-burning, fat-melting workout. Follow the program, and you're virtually guaranteed to lose weight.

Now that I've introduced you to the basic organization of the walking workouts, let's take a closer look at what you'll be doing in each. Here's a basic breakdown.

- Warm-up
- Walking workout, with targeted stretches and/or resistance-training moves
- Cooldown
- Stretching routine
- Yoga and Pilates routine (in advanced workouts only)

First, each workout begins with a 10-minute warm-up. This is a modestly paced walk geared solely to warm up and prepare your muscles for the workout ahead. (If you're doing my Treadmill Walking workout, for example, you'll complete your 10-minute warm-up walk on the treadmill, at an easy pace, with no grade.) *The warm-up time does not count toward your total walking time for the day.* Don't skip this important step: Launching right into your workout can cause soreness or injury.

After completing your warm-up, simply follow the detailed instructions for the workout you've chosen. Where appropriate, some of the workouts begin with a few targeted stretches. Complete these before you begin walking.

Once you begin walking, you'll notice that the directions are very specific, asking you to walk for a precise number of minutes at a certain rate (usually expressed in miles per hour). The reason for this is that each workout is designed to burn a precise range of calories, so it's important that you try your best to meet these requirements. Only by doing so can you get the full benefit of the workout. (In chapter 3, I'll explain how to use a pedometer to determine your distance and walking speed.)

Most of the workouts also incorporate one or two targeted strength-training moves, such as a squat or a walking lunge. You'll find that completing these moves considerably increases the challenge of the workout. Hang in there, you can do it!

Now, you'll notice that each workout has a basic, intermediate, and advanced level. These levels correspond to the levels in my 4-month program, meaning that the workouts will be getting gradually more challenging as the weeks (and months) progress. Now, unless you've been working out consistently for an hour or more at least three times a week, I want you to start with my Month #1 Workout Program, which means that you'll be doing beginner-level walking workouts.

Finally, every workout ends with a 5-minute cooldown walk (done at one-half to one-quarter of your previous pace) followed by a short Post-Workout Stretching Routine (see page 129). Don't skip this important step! Stretching lengthens and relaxes the muscles you've just worked, decreasing any pain and stiffness and keeping you limber. It can also improve your balance and posture, decrease risk of future injury, and reduce stress. Pretty good for just a few minutes of work!

Additional Workouts to Boost the Burn

If you look again at the calendars beginning on page 57, you'll notice that my program includes workouts beyond walking. For a complete, total workout, I also want you to regularly complete my Strength-Training Workout (see page 135). This full-body workout is specially designed to tone and prepare your body for the activities you do on a daily basis, things like climbing the stairs, cleaning, getting into and out of your car, hauling groceries, and carrying your children or grandchildren around. What's more, this routine will help you build calorie-hungry muscle, but without getting bulky. And the more muscle you have, the more calories your body will burn, even when you're at rest. To truly get the lean, toned body you crave, you need to combine my walking workouts with this specially designed full-body strength-training routine.

Consider Meditation

If you follow the exercise program in this book, you're going to be burning huge amounts of calories, melting away body fat, and building lean muscle. Chances are you'll start to feel better than you have in years, maybe even decades. But there's still one aspect of your health you may be forgetting, and that's your emotional health.

According to the National Institutes of Health, 80 to 90 percent of all illnesses are caused by stress, either directly or indirectly. And while exercise can help ease your stress levels, it may not be enough on its own. That's why I recommend pairing my workout program with daily meditation.

For some people, the practice of meditating can seem a little mysterious or time-consuming. But the truth is that in its most basic form, meditation is simply an attempt to tame our minds by *being still.* Think about it: When was the last time you sat completely still for 10 to 20 minutes and didn't think about any of the pressing details in your life, didn't answer the phone, didn't even look at your e-mail? Taking a few minutes each day to sit quietly with ourselves can help us to soothe our anxieties, break habitual thought patterns, increase our energy levels, and possibly even lower blood pressure.

To try out a simple form of meditation, find a quiet place where you won't be disturbed. Sit in a comfortable position, preferably with your back straight. Close your eyes and focus your mind either on your breath or on a sound or word you silently repeat to yourself. If other thoughts intervene—and they will— allow them to float away, gently refocusing as needed. Try to meditate for 10 to 20 minutes, two times a day if possible.

While there are many different types of meditation, Transcendental Meditation (TM) has been found to be more than twice as effective at reducing stress than any other form of relaxation. TM teaches you how to completely quiet your mind. If it sounds familiar, this was the type of meditation the Beatles practiced. If you'd like to give it a try, I recommend either taking a seminar or reading one of the many books available on the topic. About 15 years ago, my mom took me to a TM seminar to learn the specific techniques, and it has truly helped me in many stressful situations.

Finally, as part of the advanced walking workouts, I'd like you to complete my Yoga and Pilates Routine, found on page 149. These two disciplines offer a wonderful complement to the work you'll be doing in your walking and strength-training workouts. Made up of specific yoga and Pilates moves I've specially chosen to round out and accompany your walking workouts, this routine is challenging, but it's oh, so worth it. These moves are tops for increasing your core strength, improving flexibility, and reducing stress and tension. I think you'll love the results!

Putting It All Together

We all work better when we have a goal. That's why I've designed my program so that you can work toward a weight-loss goal each month. But being fit and healthy is a lifestyle, not something that you do for a few weeks and then forget about. In this book, I've given you 4 months of workout calendars, plus two bonus months featuring warm-weather and cold-weather workouts. I encourage you to take advantage of all of them. This will not only ensure significant weight loss, but by the time you've completed the program, working out will have become a regular part of your life—something you don't even consider *not* doing, much like brushing your teeth each morning or washing your hair. To maintain weight loss, working out needs to be a habit, and these workouts are the easiest and safest ways I know to get into that habit.

As I mentioned earlier, if you haven't been working out consistently for an hour or more at least three times a week, start out with my Month #1 Workout Program. This program will safely ease you into a regular workout program by creating a base of regularly completed basic-level workouts. Don't be fooled into thinking they won't be challenging or won't burn tons of calories, however. These are not your grandmother's walking routines! You'll still be on course for significant weight loss in your first month, but you'll do so without risking injury or soreness.

Over the next few months, you'll be increasing the challenge by completing intermediate-level and, gradually, advanced-level workouts. These are the ultimate for calorie burn and weight loss. And because you've built up a base of fitness in the preceding weeks, you'll be able to do them safely and effectively.

Of course, if you have been working out consistently for an extended period of time, feel free to skip ahead to my Month #2 Workout Program. This way, you'll be able to jump right in to workouts that are challenging for your fitness level.

Because flexibility is the name of the game in my exercise program, I've included two special months of workouts—one for warm weather and one for cold weather. Since I've lived in areas of the country that have very cold winters or very hot and humid summers, I know what weather challenges can do to your workout plans (not to mention your motivation!). That's why I've created these two unique workout programs. The warm-weather program will allow you to take advantage of the beautiful weather with lots of outdoor workouts, including one on the beach. Plus, you'll focus on workouts geared toward warm-weather activities, such as golfing and camping. And when the weather turns frigid, you can turn to my cold-weather program, which is heavy on indoor workouts, such as my Treadmill Walking workout and the Mall and Museum Walks. On those days when the sun does warm up things a bit, though, don't forget to take advantage of my Winter Wonderland program; you'll be glad you did!

Finally, at the end of this book, you'll find Walking Logs that I encourage you to fill out each and every time you work out. By closely tracking your progress, you'll be able to see how far you've come, where you still have room for improvement, and what obstacles have been getting in the way of your exercise routine. Knowledge is power, and I find that the few minutes it takes to fill out this log after every workout is time well spent.

If these directions seem pretty straightforward, it's because they are. Life is complicated enough without a complex workout program. The programs in this book are designed to be effective, fun, *and* easy to use. Enjoy their flexibility—and revel in their results!

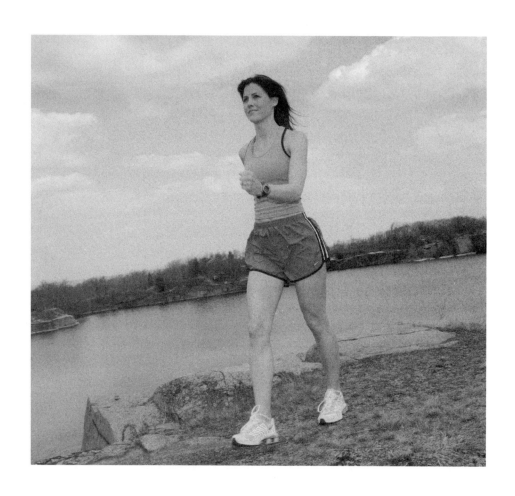

Happily may I walk.
May it be beautiful before me.
May it be beautiful behind me.
May it be beautiful below me.
May it be beautiful above me.
May it be beautiful all around me.

—Anonymous, Native American

CHAPTER THREE

Getting Started

EVERY YEAR, MILLIONS OF US pack ourselves and our families into cars, planes, or trains and head to our favorite vacation destinations; some of us head to the beach, others to theme parks, and still others to national parks, historic landmarks, or favorite cities. Regardless of our destinations, though, we all have some pre-planning to do before our vacations can begin: First, we check out maps and plot out the best routes to take, estimating how long our fun journeys will take us. Once we know how much time we'll need, we talk to our employers and schedule some time off from work. And last, we gather and pack up all the items we'll need for the journeys before heading out for our highly anticipated destinations.

Starting a walking program is much the same. You will be going on a journey with the ultimate destination of weight loss and physical fitness. But before you can head out, you need to do a little advance planning. If you've read chapter 2, you already have the "maps" you'll need to work safely and effectively through the walking program in this book. As for getting an "all clear," in this case, it needs to come from your doctor rather than your employer. Once you've gotten that, the only remaining things to do are to brush up on your basics and then gather up a few inexpensive items you'll need to complete the workouts. To get started with your preparation, read on.

Before You Walk, Have a Talk

You already walk (at least a little bit!) every day, so you may be wondering if it's really necessary to clear your new walking program with your doctor. The truth is, the walking routines in this book are challenging, and if you have certain medical conditions, you should consult your doctor by phone or in person before beginning any exercise program, including this one. For a simple quiz to determine your readiness to begin an exercise program, see page 36.

The Physical Activity Readiness Quiz

For most people, starting an exercise program is one of the healthiest things they'll do in their lives. However, if you have certain medical conditions, you should consult your doctor before beginning any exercise program, including the one in this book.

Answer yes or no to each of the following questions.

YES	NO	
☐	☐	1. Have you had your heart health checked by your doctor recently?
☐	☐	2. Have you had your blood pressure checked lately?
☐	☐	3. Do you have any medical conditions that your doctor feels would be made worse with exercise, such as dizziness, bone or joint problems, or age-related illness?

If you answered yes to one or more of the above questions, consult with your doctor before beginning this or any exercise program.

If you answered no to all of these questions and have your doctor's okay, your present condition is most likely suitable for exercise. If at any time you begin to experience any of the symptoms mentioned in the above questions, however, stop exercising and seek immediate medical assistance.

If you've been sedentary or have certain medical conditions, such as an increased risk for heart disease or stroke, I recommend that you talk with your doctor about taking a stress test before beginning the walking program. The test tells you and your doctor how well your heart can handle exercise. When you take a stress test, you're first hooked up to equipment that monitors your heart. Then you're asked to begin by walking slowly on a treadmill. Over the course of the test, the speed will be increased and the treadmill set at a small incline. During the test, your doctor will monitor your breathing, heart rate, blood pressure, and electrocardiogram. You can stop at any time, should you feel you need to.

Finally, if you have arthritis or any problems with your knees or hips, be sure to discuss this with your doctor before beginning the walking program in this book. It's very likely your doctor will tell you that the low-impact exercise you'll be getting will actually help prevent pain and further degeneration in these areas.

Finding Your Stride

Now that you've gotten your doctor's approval to start an exercise program, it's important to spend a few moments thinking about your walking mechanics. Walking truly is elegant in its simplicity, yet that doesn't mean that there aren't certain things you can do to boost the benefits you get as you walk. And paying attention to your walking stride can prevent the few injuries that sometimes do plague walkers.

Have you ever seen someone who walks on their heels? They tend to have a very rigid stride and "heavy"-sounding steps. Not only is this not the most efficient way to walk, but it can also lead to what's known as repetitive-stress injuries (injuries caused by doing the same action over and over again with improper form).

Though we almost never take the time to think about it, each step we take really consists of three separate parts: foot landing, planting, and push-off. Perhaps an easier way to think about this as you're walking, though, is to remember the mantra "Roll from heel to toe." You want to land on your heel (the foot landing step), roll your foot from heel to toe (planting), and then push off with your toes (push-off).

Here are some other tips.

Walk tall. Stand up straight as you walk—no swaybacks! Keep your shoulders down, back, and relaxed—not hunched over or rounded. Elongate your spine by looking forward, not down, as you walk. Try to gaze about 10 feet ahead of you. Your chin should be level and your head up.

Tighten your abs. As you walk, contract your abs. This keeps you from arching your lower back. Tilt your pelvis slightly forward.

Bend your arms. Keep your elbows bent at slightly less than 90-degree angles. Swing your arms front to back (not side to side), with your hands swinging in an arc from your waistband to chest height. Your arms should not cross your body. When you swing your arms fast, your feet will follow.

Push off with your toes. Concentrate on landing on your heel, rolling through the step, and then pushing off with your toes.

Pay attention to your breathing. You want to walk fast enough that your breathing is increased. Remember to breathe in through your nose and out through your mouth.

Pick up your pace properly. Don't force your stride length; let it come naturally. To go faster, take smaller, more rapid steps; don't elongate your stride. If you take 130 steps per minute (which you can determine by using a pedometer, more on that to come), you'll be walking at a pace of about 4 miles per hour, which gives you a great cardiorespiratory challenge.

Walking Precautions

Remember: For safety and effectiveness, you need to have good walking mechanics, which usually means it's best to keep your workouts simple. On that note, here are a few things to avoid.

Ankle weights: Wearing ankle weights as you do your walking routine can place excessive stress on the ligaments of your ankles and knees. This creates an unnatural walking pattern, which can lead to pain in the ankles, knees, and lower back. Ankle weights should be used only for exercises that keep you in a fixed position.

Hand weights: It's best to leave the hand weights at home, too. Any benefit you could get from using them is overshadowed by the risks. Their additional weight imposes unnecessary forces on the wrists, elbows, shoulders, neck, and lower back. The physical adjustments you must make to maintain the stability of the hand weights aren't conducive to a healthy, productive exercise session. The walking programs in this book will teach you how to add intensity to your workouts safely, without the use of weights.

Exercising in extreme heat or cold: The physical adaptations that your body must endure to maintain and regulate body temperature under extreme conditions require your cardiovascular system to work overtime. Adding the workload of exercise to this equation can be dangerous. When the day is expected to be a scorcher, try working out as early as possible in the morning, when temperatures should be at their coolest. Or do a treadmill workout indoors or a workout at the mall when the weather outside isn't cooperating with your workout goals.

Your Essential Walking "Equipment"

The final step before you begin the walking program is to make sure you're properly outfitted for the journey ahead. You wouldn't head out to the beach without your bathing suit, would you? Likewise, you want to make sure you have the proper equipment before you get started on your walking program. Fortunately, you won't need much gear, but making sure that the few items you do need are well made and fit comfortably can make a big difference in the amount of enjoyment you get out of your walks. And when it comes to picking shoes, choosing the right style can actually reduce your risk of injury.

These Shoes Were Made for Walkin'

If you haven't been in an athletic shoe store for a while, you'll probably be surprised by the number of different types and styles of what used to just be called "sneakers." Today, there are specialty shoes for nearly any activity you're planning to do—including basketball, tennis, and even volleyball! There are also specialty shoes for walking and running. In general, I think that running shoes work best for runners *and* walkers. The gait pattern of the foot is the same for both activities, and there's a much greater selection of running shoes to fit your foot type, level of fitness, and terrain of choice.

And speaking of terrain, one of the first things to consider when looking for your new shoes is where you'll be taking them. If you plan to spend a lot of your walking time off-road—such as walking on trails in parks, wooded areas, or fields—you'll want a shoe that has a reinforced midsole (the part of the shoe between the outer sole, which touches the ground, and the shoe upper) that can withstand the additional strain of this uneven terrain. And because when you're off-road, you're much more likely to deal with what exercise physiologists call "lateral instability"—the side-to-side instability that can make you roll your ankle—you'll want to find a shoe with extra support and a more aggressive tread.

After thinking about the places you'll be wearing your shoes, the next factor to consider is your foot shape. Shoes are formed on a mold called a last. There are three basic types of lasts, and they produce three basic shapes of shoes: straight, semi-curved, and curved. You'll want to choose the shoe type that matches the shape of your feet.

Shoes made on *straight* lasts are designed for people with flat feet. If you flip the shoe over, you'll see that the shoe barely, if at all, curves from the heel to the toe box (the part of the shoe that, as the name suggests, encases your toes). The sole of this shoe will be broad and about the same width from the heel through the midfoot.

Shoes formed on *semi-curved* lasts are designed for people with mid-height arches, which is the majority of the population. These shoes have a slight curvature from heel to toe. The sole of this shoe is wider at the heel and then narrows slightly toward midfoot.

And finally, shoes made on *curved* lasts are ideal for people with high arches. If you flip this shoe over, you'll notice that it's not nearly as wide at the midfoot as it is at the heel. In fact, if you follow the line of the shoe from the heel to the toes, you'll see that it mimics the curvature of the letter "s."

Matching the shape of your shoe to the shape of your foot is more than just an issue of comfort. Wearing an improperly fitting shoe can actually increase your risk for injury. For example, suppose you have flat feet, but you put on a pair of running shoes with significant arch support (what's known in shoe company lingo as "medial posting"). These shoes will cause your feet to lean outward, making it difficult for you to complete a neutral stride. Not only will these shoes feel uncomfortable, but wearing them can throw your body out of alignment, causing problems with your knees, hips, and spine. The inverse goes for people with high-arched feet. If they wear shoes without arch support, they'll likely overpronate, which means their ankles will be rolling inward as they walk. Overpronation causes excessive stress first on the plantar fascia (the broad band of fibrous tissue that runs along the bottom of the foot), and then upward to the knees and hips.

After determining which of the three shoe shapes is right for you, you'll want to consider shoe width. Most of us have medium-width feet, give or take a few millimeters, but for folks with narrower or wider feet, there are three to four widths available from most of the major shoe companies.

Here are a few more tips for finding the perfect shoe for you.

Shop for shoes in the afternoon or evening. Everyone's feet swell during the course of the day, so it's important to do your shoe shopping toward the end of the day, when your feet are at their largest. Otherwise, you might end up with shoes that are too small.

Wear or bring along your workout socks. The thickness of your socks can drastically change the way your shoes fit, so be sure to try on shoes while wearing the socks you'll be donning to do your walking workouts. It really does make a difference.

Go to the experts. Always go to a specialty shoe store, preferably one that's individually owned. Chain stores don't train their employees in the exquisite art of shoe fitting; instead, their focus seems to be on selling you whatever happens to be the latest "hot," trendy shoe. I've seen customers walk into these types of stores asking for running shoes and walk out with new pairs of orange Converse basketball shoes! Avoid the marketing hype and stick with the advice of the experts.

Expect to be asked some questions. If the salesperson doesn't ask you at least the following questions, you're in the wrong place.

- How often do you walk?
- Would you take off your shoes so we can look at and measure your feet?
- Do you wear orthotics?
- Do you have any foot, knee, or hip injuries or limitations?

Take a stroll. After you and the salesperson have selected a few different pairs of shoes that fit your needs, take the time to walk around in each of them. Don't let yourself be hurried; this is an important step that too many people rush through. Likewise, don't be afraid to try on lots of different pairs of shoes. This is the only way you can find the ones that fit you best.

Consider the fit. The shoes should fit like a glove, never too tight nor loose enough to let your foot slide around. Shoes will stretch a bit over time, so keep that in mind. Make sure the shoe fits the contours of your foot, especially in the

A Word about Water (And Other Drinks)

In chapter 1, I briefly discussed the importance of drinking water throughout the day as part of an overall diet plan. But when you begin an intense workout program such as the one in this book, taking in lots of fluids becomes even more important. Staying well hydrated allows your muscles to contract more easily and to flush out the metabolic wastes produced during exercise. It also makes your blood less viscous, allowing it be pumped throughout your body with less resistance, creating a lower resting blood pressure. Most important, it helps your body to cool itself and keep blood flowing through it at a stable temperature.

While the minimum recommended amount of water you should take in daily is 64 ounces per day, or about 8 glasses, this figure doesn't take into account the fluids you lose when you complete a hard workout. So make 64 ounces per day your bare minimum and be sure to get even more than that on the days you work out. And, of course, pay special attention to staying hydrated during particularly warm days.

During exercise, I find it's best to drink cold fluids, rather than room-temperature ones. Cold fluids seem to satisfy the body better, and they taste better, which means you'll drink more. The best fluids to drink during exercise are water, sports energy drinks, and diluted fruit juice. These drinks are tops both for hydration and for replacing the electrolytes that are depleted during vigorous exercise.

I recommend wearing a fanny pack during your walks and using it to store your water bottles. That way, your hands can remain free, but you'll always have a drink ready to sip from frequently.

mid- and rear foot, with just enough room for your forefoot to lay flat, with your toes relaxed. You should not feel any pressure in your toes.

Ask about orthotics. Orthotics are designed to create a healthy landing pattern for the foot, complementing the existing structures of your shoes. They can enhance your foot's stability, while allowing a proper, neutral gait pattern, thereby reducing any unnecessary strain on your knees and hips. There are now several types of orthotics available over the counter; you simply place them inside your athletic shoes. If you think an orthotic might be helpful for you, visit a podiatrist or speak to your local shoe-fitting expert.

Monitor your shoes for signs of wear. Your shoes are all that come between you and your walking surface, so it's important to replace them when they become worn. To determine if it's time for a new pair, place your old shoes on a table or other flat surface and take a look at them from the back. If they lean inward or outward or show signs of excessive wear, such as soles with badly worn edges, it's probably time for a new pair. Even if your shoes look like they're in good shape, it may be time to replace them if you've logged 500 or more miles in them or if you start to notice pain in your feet, ankles, legs, or knees even though you haven't changed your exercise routine.

After you buy new shoes, go to the store and try on a new pair of that same model about every 4 to 6 months, depending on the amount of walking you're doing. You may not realize how much your shoes have worn until you try on a new pair.

Having happy feet can mean so much for an exercise program. We walk from the ground up. If all is right at the foundation, we can expect similar results throughout the rest of our bodies. Our exercise routines will continue and our progress will, too.

Socks: Keeping Your Feet Dry and Happy

They may seem like a minor item, but the socks you choose can make a huge difference in your comfort level during your workouts. Look for performance socks, which are typically made of a polyester blend. What's wrong with cotton? It holds 20 times more moisture than these new fabrics. All that moisture can cause your feet to become damp with sweat, which can increase bacterial production—definitely not the healthiest environment for your feet! Plus, moisture can cause the sock to bunch, creating pressure points in your walking shoes and leading to blisters.

Performance socks wick away moisture, keeping your feet dry and healthy. There are several different blends of synthetic socks that you can choose from; some even have elastic worked into the midfoot to add support. Another popular choice for winter walks is socks made of merino wool, which are known for their snug fit, long life, and all-around comfort.

Note: To minimize the friction that can cause blisters, rub a thin layer of petroleum jelly on areas particularly prone to them (i.e., your heels, the side of your baby toe). Also, consider using a foot powder or antiperspirant to keep your feet dry.

Apparel: Style and Comfort

Although you don't need to invest in a whole new wardrobe for your walking workouts, I do suggest that you purchase a few quality pieces. Today's athletic apparel is designed to keep you dry and comfortable whether it's 5 degrees or 85 degrees outside. Look for clothes made with a polyester blend of materials called Coolmax. It's the latest and greatest in athletic apparel technology. Coolmax fabric is specially designed to quickly move moisture away from the skin to the outer layer of the fabric. It then dries the moisture faster than any other fabric available today.

If it's cold where you live and you plan on doing some of my outdoor workouts, you'll want to dress in layers. Nearest to your skin, you'll want to wear clothing made of Coolmax or other moisture-wicking fabric. Then, depending on the temperature, you'll need to add layers of fleece or wool. Finally, top it all off with a wind-resistant jacket or coat, some gloves, and a hat.

If you plan to do some or all of your walking in the evenings, you'll need to add some reflective gear to your workout wardrobe. See "Walk Safely" on page 44 for my recommendations.

Finally, because you'll be adding in various exercises at timed intervals during your walks, be sure to wear a watch I like the watches that offer features that include heart rate monitors, stopwatch, and calorie expenditure. For long walks I also recommend wearing a fanny pack, which will allow you to easily carry your water, some cash, and your cell phone.

Pedometers: The Easiest Way to Measure Distance

Pedometers measure the distance you walk by counting each step you take. You wear them on your hip, and they work by counting up the number of times you move your leg to take a step. To calculate the distance you've traveled, the pedometer will multiply the number of steps you've taken by your stride length (which you need to input before using the pedometer, more on that shortly). Because many of the walking workouts in this book require you to walk for a specific distance or at a specific speed, you'll need to use a pedometer.

Walk Safely

Both of my sisters enjoy walking outdoors for exercise. My younger sister, Nicole, lives in Vail, Colorado, and she often walks in the mountains surrounding her house. Nik occasionally finds herself on mountainous roads where cars speed around the corners with little notice. Similarly, my older sister, Michele, walks with friends and their children in Canyon Lake, Texas. Michele says, "I can't always avoid traffic to and from the lake."

I recently sent both my sisters reflective vests, ankle strips, and reflective tape to place on their shoes, bikes, or strollers. (I'm currently working with Graco to add a reflective strip to their jogging strollers.) Nicole has gone a step further by adding a safety light to her headband for winter evenings—mostly because of the deer that seem to jump out of nowhere.

To ensure that your own outings are safe and pleasurable, take these steps.

Face the traffic. If you're walking on the road, always walk facing oncoming traffic. Drivers at night or in the early mornings are rarely on the lookout for walkers.

Color me safe. For workouts at dusk or dawn (and anytime on cloudy, dark days), wear light-colored clothing. The worst colors to wear at these times are blue (especially navy) and black, which make you virtually invisible to traffic. White, orange, and yellow are the easiest colors to see.

Reflect your presence. You can purchase light sticks, luminous tape (which you can put on your shoes, clothing, bike, stroller, etc.), and reflective vests, gloves, and headbands online at www.reflexsafety.com. You can also find these products at most fitness and department stores. Both Nike and Adidas make great reflective jackets, bike shorts, and tops.

Leave jewelry at home. The only accessories you need are a wristwatch or stopwatch.

Bring your ID. Always carry some form of identification in case of an accident or medical emergency—and maybe a small amount of cash.

Prepare for allergies. If you have allergies, also be sure to tuck your doctor-prescribed EpiPen into your pocket. More than one pleasant walk through a field covered in wildflowers has been interrupted by a confrontation with an angry bee.

Try not to walk alone. If at all possible, walk with a training partner. Not only does this increase your safety while walking, but it also makes your training so much more enjoyable. If your training partner is a four-legged friend, let someone know where you're going and what time you expect to return.

Take along your cell. If you're the type of person who often decides to change your route midwalk, a cell phone can come in handy to let the folks back home know where you'll be. Wearing a fanny pack gives you a convenient place to hold your cell phone as well as water.

Leave the mp3 at home. I'm amazed at runners, walkers, and cyclists who think they can hear surrounding noises while they're pumping music into their ears. To stay safe, you need to be able to hear things like dogs, cars, horns, other people, and thunder.

Vary your route. Mix up your routes and the time that you go out to walk. Not only is it safer (some attackers have confessed to watching victims in the days prior to an attack to determine their routines), but any time you change the route your walk, it can be more challenging for your muscles and more interesting for your mind.

Think self-defense. Whether I'm walking in New York City's Central Park at dawn or on the highly traveled beach paths near my home in Connecticut, I always carry my hand-held spray mace. These devices are designed to fit comfortably in your hand, are very light, and are easy to use. You can purchase mace online or at any security store.

You can purchase a pedometer at any sporting goods store and in some large discount stores. For our workouts, you won't need a fancy model, but I do recommend purchasing one that automatically calculates the distance you've traveled and tells you your walking speed. Other than that, be aware that higher-priced models offer additional features, but they aren't required for the workouts you'll be doing in this book. For example, fancy ones have timers, stopwatches, and a week's worth of memory, so you can store your workout results.

Before you can begin using your pedometer, you need to determine your stride length. To do this, take 10 normal steps from a set starting point. After your 10th step, use chalk or tape to mark the point where the front of your forward foot hits the ground. Then measure the distance you've traveled and divide by 10 to get your stride length. For example, if your total distance is 20 feet, your stride length is 2 feet. Then follow the manufacturer's instructions to input your stride length. You're now set to begin using your pedometer.

Beyond using pedometers to calculate distance during your walking workouts, they can also be a great motivational tool to increase your activity level throughout the day. That's why I'd like to recommend that you wear a pedometer all day long, especially on the days when you're not scheduled for a walking workout. (For the results of an intriguing study on the use of pedometers, see "For Added Incentive, Wear a Pedometer" on page 47.) Simply wear your pedometer from the time you get up until the time you turn in for the night. Before you hop into bed, record the total number of steps you took that day in your Walking Log (see page 161). You can play a game with yourself to try to increase the number of steps you take each day. You'll be surprised how many more steps you can incorporate into your day by making simple lifestyle modifications such as parking your car farther away from the store, taking the time to play active games with your kids, walking to your coworker's desk instead of sending an e-mail, and so on.

Note: Incorrect placement of your pedometer may result in only a portion of your steps being counted. To count steps accurately, your pedometer needs to hang vertically from your your waist and be aligned over your knee. Clip your pedometer to the waistband of your pants (or a pocket just below the waistband) to make sure it's counting all of your strides.

StrengthTraining with Physioballs and Exercise Bands

As I discussed in chapter 2, you'll also be doing a targeted strength-training routine a number of times each week in addition to your walking workouts. To complete this routine, you'll need a physioball (also known as a Swiss ball, fitness ball, or stability ball) and an exercise band.

Physioballs

Most resistance training exercises work only one joint at a time, in a single plane of motion. But our day-to-day activities require us to move in multiple planes, using numerous muscles and joints at once. How can we increase the challenge of our workouts to address this need? A physioball.

Because these oversized rubber balls provide an unstable surface, they make your workout session more challenging. To perform exercises using one, you need to use multiple muscle groups at once, which increases your balance, coordination, and mobility. You'll also improve your awareness of your joint and body position as you work out, since you'll need to make continual adjustments to maintain proper balance.

For Added Incentive, Wear a Pedometer

According to doctors, each of us should get at least 30 minutes of exercise a day, which if walking is your exercise of choice amounts to about 10,000 steps. Yet although that's a bare minimum, many of us don't get even that much exercise. Often, the problem is as simple as a lack of motivation. Fortunately, there may be an equally simple answer: wearing a pedometer.

In a recent study, Dixie L. Thompson, Ph.D., and her colleagues at the University of Tennessee studied what effect wearing a pedometer might have on the motivation levels of 58 middle-aged women. Before the study, none of the women got much exercise; they averaged only 5,760 steps per day. Perhaps as a result, all of the women were overweight or obese.

Dr. Thompson and her colleagues broke the women into two groups. They told the first group to "take a brisk 30-minute walk on most, or preferably all, days of the week." The women were given pedometers so that the researchers could record how many steps they actually took. However, the pedometers were sealed, so that the women themselves couldn't read their number of steps.

The researchers told the second group of women to walk 10,000 steps a day. These women were also given a sealed pedometer, but in addition, they were given another pedometer that showed them how many steps they took each day.

The first group of women (those who were told to take a 30-minute walk but were given only sealed pedometers) averaged about 10,000 steps, but only on those days when they actually took a walk. On the remaining days, they tended to sit around as usual.

In contrast, the second group of women (those who were told to walk 10,000 steps every day and were given pedometers they could read) averaged 12,000 steps on days they went for a walk. Yet even on those days when they didn't go out walking, they still increased their daily number of steps to about 8,000.

According to Dr. Thompson, the study shows that pedometers can be a great incentive for people to increase their daily activity levels. If you sometimes find it hard to get off the couch and start walking, wearing a pedometer throughout the day might be just the incentive you need. This can be especially helpful on the days you aren't scheduled to do a walking workout from this book. Simply put on the pedometer in the morning and don't take it off until you go to bed at night. Record your number of steps in your Walking Log, and then each day try to increase that number.

If you don't have a physioball, you can purchase one at most sporting goods stores, many discount superstores, and even online. They sell for about $25, and they come in four sizes. The right size for you depends on your height.

If you're...	Choose a Physioball That Measures...
Less than 5'0"	45 centimeters (18 inches)
5'0" to 5'6"	55 centimeters (22 inches)
5'7" to 6'1"	65 centimeters (26 inches)
6'2" to 6'8"	75 centimeters (30 inches)
6'9" and up	85 centimeters (34 inches)

You'll want to maintain a neutral pelvic posture during core/trunk exercises performed on a physioball. Also, always wear rubber-soled shoes for traction, avoid bouncing on the ball while bending or twisting your spine, and be sure to perform exercises slowly and with body control. Roll on and off the ball slowly and have someone spot you for the more challenging exercises.

Exercise Bands

Exercise bands are flat bands made of rubber tubing. They come in different resistance levels, which are distinguished by the color of the band. The band you should use depends on your strength level, height (the taller you are, the more the band stretches, so the harder the exercise is), and the type of exercise you'll be doing with it.

Because exercise bands are so light and portable, they're ideal for travelers. Simply tuck them in your suitcase, and you're all set for a great workout in your hotel room. Another advantage of exercise bands is that you can vary the tension as you use the band to make an exercise easier or more difficult. You can also do exercises with them that can't be done with free weights or machines. And finally, if you're doing multifunctional exercises, such as balance exercises or working out on a physioball, exercise bands are easier to hold than free weights.

My favorite exercise bands are made by Perform Better. You can contact them by logging on to www.performbetter.com or calling (888) 556-7464. You can also buy exercise bands at most major sporting goods stores.

Heart Rate Monitors

Although you don't absolutely have to have a heart rate monitor to complete the exercise program in this book, I do recommend investing in one because they're

Get in the Zone

How do you know if you're working out hard enough, but not so hard that you risk injury? One of the most accurate ways is to monitor your heart rate using something called the *target heart rate zone.* Keeping your heart rate within this zone ensures that your exercise intensity isn't so high that it's counterproductive or even dangerous, and that it isn't so low that you're not getting any health benefits. Using this approach requires measuring your pulse periodically as you exercise—a task that's made much easier with a heart rate monitor. Your goal is to stay within 50 to 75 percent of your maximum heart rate.

Your *maximum heart rate* is the greatest number of times per minute that your heart is capable of beating. On average, it can be determined by subtracting your age from 220. You never want to work out at this rate, though. Instead, you want to work out at about 50 to 75 percent of it, which scientists have determined is a safe but effective intensity level.

To determine your target heart rate zone, use the following simple formula.

Target Heart Rate = Maximum Heart Rate X Percent Intensity

First, figure out your Maximum Heart Rate and write it here:

220 – Your Age = _____

Now, to find the low end of your target heart rate zone,
multiply your Maximum Heart Rate by 0.50 (or 50 percent): _____

To find the high end of your target heart rate zone,
multiply your Maximum Heart Rate by 0.75 (or 75 percent): _____

For example, if you're 40 years old, your maximum heart rate would be 180 (220 – 40 = 180). The low end of your target heart rate zone would be 50 percent of 180, or 90. The high end of your target heart rate zone would be 75 percent of 180, or 135.

For a safe, effective workout, you'd want to try to keep your heart rate within the 90 to 135 beats per minute zone for the duration of the workout. (Always warm up first, though, and follow your workout with a cooldown walk at one-half to one-quarter of your previous pace, as directed in the workouts in part two of this book.)

such helpful tools. (Plus, you'll be able to do my Heart Healthy workout more easily if you have a monitor.) A heart rate monitor can help you make sure you're working at an effective pace—not so high that your workout becomes counterproductive or even dangerous, and not so low that you don't gain benefits. While there are more complicated monitors designed for elite athletes that provide an array of detailed fitness information, the most basic monitors simply sense and display the number of times your heart is beating per minute (bpm). Slightly more expensive models allow you to set the monitor to give you a warning beep when your heart rate drops below or speeds ahead of your *target* heart rate zone, which I'll explain next. That way, you can adjust your intensity to get the best workout. The most accurate monitors are designed to be strapped tightly around the chest. The information is then sent to a display, which is usually worn like a wristwatch. With other varieties of monitors, you forgo the chest strap and instead place one or two fingers on sensor buttons, giving you an "on demand," rather than constant, reading. Still other varieties use ear clips.

Before you can use a heart rate monitor, you need to determine your target heart rate zone. To do this, see "Get in the Zone."

Once you've determined your target heart rate zone, staying within it becomes much easier with a heart rate monitor. Of course, you can also monitor your heart rate the old-fashioned way: by simply finding your pulse and counting the number of beats per minute. (I find it easiest to count the number of beats for 10 seconds, then multiply by 6.) But for people who find working with technology motivating, heart rate monitors can be just the ticket to get them up and moving.

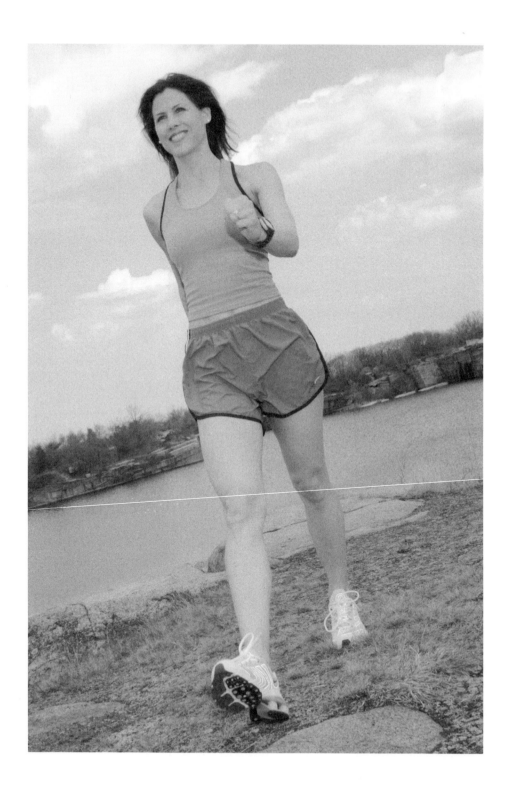

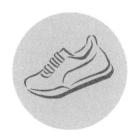

PART TWO

The Walk-Off-
the-Weight
Exercise Program

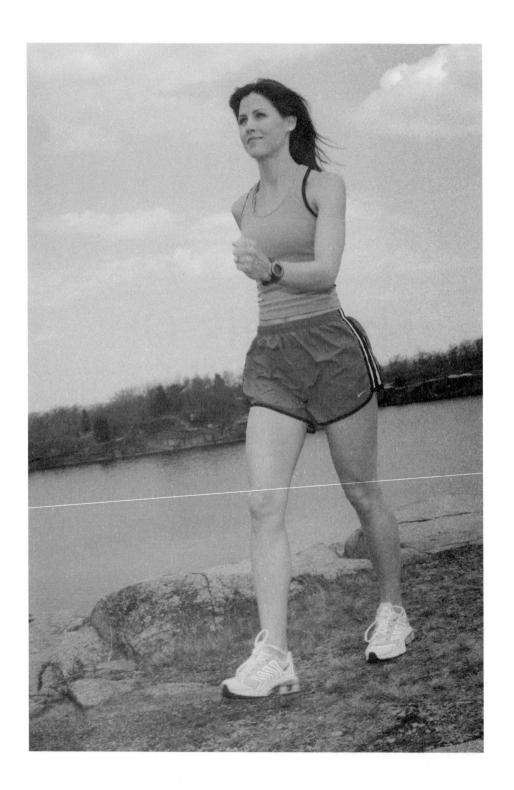

CHAPTER FOUR

The 4-Month Program

FOLLOWING ARE THE CALENDARS for my 4-month program, which gets progressively more challenging with each month, plus two bonus months for specialized workouts depending on the weather.

As you'll see, I've taken the guesswork out of my exercise program. Simply follow the plan, and you're guaranteed to lose weight and feel better. But I also understand that life happens. Schedules are unpredictable, you may be asked to take a business trip at the last moment, or you might have special needs you're looking to address, such as arthritis pain or high cholesterol. Whatever situation you find yourself in, there's a workout in this book you can do. If one of the suggested workouts for that day doesn't fit in with your plans, simply substitute another one from part two of this book. The only stipulation is that I'd like you to try *not* to do the same workout more than twice in one week. Remember: Your body gets strongest when you're constantly throwing new challenges at it, so doing a variety of workouts each week will give you the best results.

Likewise, if I've scheduled a walking workout for, say, Wednesday, but you're unable to fit it in that day, you can move that workout to another day in the same week. I do want you to be sure, though, that you get in the number of workouts I've planned for that week. And to give your muscles proper time to rest and rebuild, try not to do the strength-training workout on consecutive days.

If you haven't been working out consistently for an hour or more at least three times a week, start out with my Month #1 Workout Program. By completing a base level of easier workouts, you'll prepare your body for the challenges of the intermediate and advanced workouts in months 2 and 3. If you have been working out consistently for an extended period of time, go ahead and start with my Month #2 Workout Program, which is challenging even for an experienced exerciser.

My optional Warm-Weather and Cold-Weather Workout Programs were built around the concept of flexibility. I've lived in many parts of the country, including New York City, where winters can get very cold, and Dallas and Atlanta, where summers can get very hot and humid so I know how hard it can be to stick to a rigid exercise program when the weather isn't cooperating. With that in mind, I've devoted these months to seasonal workouts. Consider it a bonus if you live in an area that's warm all the time, such as California or Florida. You can head right to the warm-weather workouts no matter what time of the year it is.

If you choose to do the Warm-Weather or Cold-Weather Workout Programs, simply do the workouts as suggested within either of these programs, at the appropriate level—beginner, intermediate, or advanced—for you. So, for example, if you're just starting my workout program and haven't been exercising regularly up to now, but it's the middle of the summer and you want to take advantage of the Warm-Weather Workout Program, follow that program as directed, doing all of the workouts at the beginner level. Once the month is over, you can move ahead to the Month #2 Workout Program. On the other hand, suppose it's the dead of winter and you've already worked through the first 3 months of the program and are ready for the advanced workouts. You now have the option to either complete Month #4 of the 4-month program or substitute the Cold-Weather Workout Program, doing all of the workouts in that program at the advanced level. Finally, if you've completed all 4 months and are looking for new ways to expand your exercise program, try out the Warm-Weather or Cold-Weather Workout Program, as appropriate depending on the calendar and where you live, completing the workouts in that program at the advanced level.

Month #1 Workout Program

Though this is my beginner-level program, most people will still find it challenging. During this month, you'll be walking 5 days a week and completing my Strength-Training Workout on the remaining 2 days. If you are beginning this exercise program after having surgery, or if you are a new mom, you can substitute my Post-Pregnancy or Post-Surgery Workout for any of the workouts listed here.

If your business or vacation plans take you away from home during this month, complete my Business and Vacation Travel workout on page 111, beginner level, instead of the suggested workout for that day. And if the day turns out to be cold and snowy, substitute the suggested workout with the Winter Wonderland workout, beginner level, on page 120.

Week #1

MONDAY	Exploring Your Neighborhood, *beginner level* (page 85) **OR** Treadmill Walking, *beginner level* (page 87)
TUESDAY	Strength-Training Workout, *beginner level* (page 135)
WEDNESDAY	Walking for Work, *beginner level* (page 90) **OR** Walking for the Fairway, *beginner level* (page 98)
THURSDAY	Strength-Training Workout, *beginner level* (page 135)
FRIDAY	Now and Later, *beginner level* (page 103) **OR** No Joint Pain Necessary, *beginner level* (page 108)
SATURDAY	Walking for Work, *beginner level* (page 90) **OR** Walking for the Fairway, *beginner level* (page 98)
SUNDAY	Exploring Your Neighborhood, *beginner level* (page 85) **OR** Treadmill Walking, *beginner level* (page 87) **OR** Mall and Museum Walks, *beginner level* (page 93)

Week #2

MONDAY	Heart Healthy, *beginner level* (page 105) **OR** Walking for Work, *beginner level* (page 90)
TUESDAY	Strength-Training Workout, *beginner level* (page 135)
WEDNESDAY	Treadmill Walking, *beginner level* (page 87) **OR** The Great Outdoors Workout #1, *beginner level* (page 99)
THURSDAY	Exploring Your Neighborhood, *beginner level* (page 85) **OR** No Joint Pain Necessary, *beginner level* (page 108)
FRIDAY	Now and Later, *beginner level* (page 103) **OR** Mall and Museum Walks, *beginner level* (page 93) **OR** Baby, Stroller, and You, *beginner level* (page 117)
SATURDAY	Strength-Training Workout, *beginner level* (page 135)
SUNDAY	Heart Healthy, *beginner level* (page 105) **OR** Walking for Work, *beginner level* (page 90) **OR** Treadmill Walking, *beginner level* (page 87)

Week #3

MONDAY	No Joint Pain Necessary, *beginner level* (page 108) **OR** Hit the Beach! *beginner level* (page 119)
TUESDAY	Strength-Training Workout, *beginner level* (page 135)
WEDNESDAY	Exploring Your Neighborhood, *beginner level* (page 85) **OR** Treadmill Walking, *beginner level* (page 87) **OR** Business and Vacation Travel, *beginner level* (page 111)
THURSDAY	Strength-Training Workout, *beginner level* (page 135)
FRIDAY	Walking for Work, *beginner level* (page 90) **OR** The Great Outdoors, Workout #1, *beginner level* (page 99)
SATURDAY	The Interval Workout, *beginner level* (page 97) **OR** Mall and Museum Walks, *beginner level* (page 93)
SUNDAY	No Joint Pain Necessary, *beginner level* (page 108) **OR** Hit the Beach! *beginner level* (page 119)

Week #4

MONDAY	Heart Healthy, *beginner level* (page 105) **OR** Treadmill Walking, *beginner level* (page 87) **OR** Walking for the Fairway, *beginner level* (page 98)
TUESDAY	Strength-Training Workout, *beginner level* (page 135)
WEDNESDAY	Now and Later, *beginner level* (page 102) **OR** The Great Outdoors, Workout #1, *beginner level* (page 99) **OR** Mall and Museum Walks, *beginner level* (page 93)
THURSDAY	Exploring Your Neighborhood, *beginner level* (page 88) **OR** No Joint Pain Necessary, *beginner level* (page 108)
FRIDAY	Interval Workout, *beginner level* (page 97) **OR** Baby, Stroller, and You, *beginner level* (page 117)
SATURDAY	Strength-Training Workout, *beginner level* (page 135)
SUNDAY	Heart Healthy, *beginner level* (page 105) **OR** Treadmill Walking, *beginner level* (page 87) **OR** Walking for the Fairway, *beginner level* (page 98)

Month #2 Workout Program

Complete the following monthly workout plan after finishing month #1 or if you were already working out consistently for an hour or more at least three times a week before picking up this book. During this month, you'll be doing either beginner- or intermediate-level walking workouts 5 days a week. On the remaining 2 days, you'll be completing my Strength-Training Workout. Note that you'll be doing the beginner version of it during the first 2 weeks, but then progressing to the intermediate version as you get stronger.

If your business or vacation plans take you away from home during this month, complete my Business and Vacation Travel workout on page 111, beginner or intermediate level, instead of the suggested workout for that day. And if the day turns out to be cold and snowy, substitute the suggested workout with the Winter Wonderland workout, beginner or intermediate level, on page 120.

Week #1

MONDAY	Treadmill Walking, *beginner level* (page 87) **OR** Exploring Your Neighborhood, *beginner level* (page 85)
TUESDAY	Strength-Training Workout, *beginner level* (page 135)
WEDNESDAY	Walking for the Fairway, *beginner level* (page 98) **OR** Interval Workout, *beginner level* (page 97)
THURSDAY	Strength-Training Workout, *beginner level* (page 135)
FRIDAY	Now and Later, *beginner level* (page 103) **OR** Heart Healthy, *beginner level* (page 105)
SATURDAY	Walking for Work, *beginner level* (page 90) **OR** Mall and Museum Walks, *beginner level* (page 93)
SUNDAY	Treadmill Walking, *beginner level* (page 87) **OR** Exploring Your Neighborhood, *beginner level* (page 85)

Week #2

MONDAY	No Joint Pain Necessary, *beginner level* (page 108) **OR** Walking for Work, *beginner level* (page 90)
TUESDAY	Strength-Training Workout, *beginner level* (page 135)
WEDNESDAY	Treadmill Walking, *beginner level* (page 87) **OR** Exploring Your Neighborhood, *beginner level* (page 87)
THURSDAY	Heart Healthy, *beginner level* (page 105) **OR** The Great Outdoors Workout #1, *intermediate level* (page 99)
FRIDAY	Now and Later, *beginner level* (page 103) **OR** Baby, Stroller, and You, *beginner level* (page 117) **OR** Treadmill Walking, *beginner level* (page 87)
SATURDAY	Strength-Training Workout, *beginner level* (page 135)
SUNDAY	No Joint Pain Necessary, *beginner level* (page 108) **OR** Walking for Work, *beginner level* (page 90) **OR** Mall and Museum Walks, *beginner level* (page 93)

Week #3

MONDAY	Heart Healthy, *intermediate level* (page 105) **OR** Hit the Beach! *intermediate level* (page 119) **OR** Treadmill Walking, *intermediate level* (page 87)
TUESDAY	Strength-Training Workout, *intermediate level* (page 135)
WEDNESDAY	No Joint Pain Necessary, *intermediate level* (page 108) **OR** Exploring Your Neighborhood, *intermediate level* (page 85)
THURSDAY	Strength-Training Workout, *intermediate level* (page 135)
FRIDAY	Walking for Work, *intermediate level* (page 90) **OR** The Great Outdoors, Workout #1, *intermediate level* (page 99)
SATURDAY	The Interval Workout, *intermediate level* (page 97) **OR** Mall and Museum Walks, *intermediate level* (page 93)
SUNDAY	Heart Healthy, *intermediate level* (page 105) **OR** Hit the Beach! *intermediate level* (page 119) **OR** Treadmill Walking, *intermediate level* (page 87)

Week #4

MONDAY	Walking for the Fairway, *intermediate level* (page 98) **OR** The Interval Workout, *intermediate level* (page 97)
TUESDAY	Strength-Training Workout, *intermediate level* (page 135)
WEDNESDAY	Now and Later, *intermediate level* (page 103) **OR** Treadmill Walking, *intermediate level* (page 87) **OR** Mall and Museum Walks, *intermediate level* (page 93)
THURSDAY	Exploring Your Neighborhood, *intermediate level* (page 85) **OR** No Joint Pain Necessary, *intermediate level* (page 108)
FRIDAY	Heart Healthy, *intermediate level* (page 105) **OR** Baby, Stroller, and You, *intermediate level* (page 117)
SATURDAY	Strength-Training Workout, *intermediate level* (page 135)
SUNDAY	Walking for the Fairway, *intermediate level* (page 98) **OR** Interval Workout, *intermediate level* (page 97) **OR** The Great Outdoors Workout #2, *beginner level* (page 101)

Month #3 Workout Program

Complete the following monthly workout plan after finishing month #2. During this month, you'll be doing either intermediate- or advanced-level walking workouts 5 days a week. On the remaining 2 days, you'll be completing my Strength-Training Workout. Note that you'll be doing the intermediate version of it during weeks 1 and 2, but then progressing to the advanced version for weeks 3 and 4.

If your business or vacation plans take you away from home during this month, complete my Business and Vacation Travel workout on page 111, intermediate or advanced level, instead of the suggested workout for that day. And if the day turns out to be cold and snowy, substitute the suggested workout with the Winter Wonderland workout, intermediate or advanced level, on page 120.

Week #1

MONDAY	Exploring Your Neighborhood, *intermediate level* (page 85) **OR** Treadmill Walking, *intermediate level* (page 87)
TUESDAY	Strength-Training Workout, *intermediate level* (page 135)
WEDNESDAY	The Interval Workout, *intermediate level* (page 97) **OR** No Joint Pain Necessary, *intermediate level* (page 108) **OR** Walking for the Fairway, *intermediate level* (page 98)
THURSDAY	Strength-Training Workout, *intermediate level* (page 135)
FRIDAY	Heart Healthy, *intermediate level* (page 105) **OR** Now and Later, *intermediate level* (page 103) **OR** The Great Outdoors Workout #1, *advanced level* (page 99)
SATURDAY	Mall and Museum Walks, *intermediate level* (page 93) **OR** Walking for Work, *intermediate level* (page 90)
SUNDAY	Exploring Your Neighborhood, *intermediate level* (page 85) **OR** Treadmill Walking, *intermediate level* (page 87) **OR** Hit the Beach! *intermediate level* (page 119)

Week #2

MONDAY	The Interval Workout, *intermediate level* (page 97) **OR** No Joint Pain Necessary, *intermediate level* (page 108) **OR** Walking for Work, *intermediate level* (page 90)
TUESDAY	Strength-Training Workout, *intermediate level* (page 135)
WEDNESDAY	Treadmill Walking, *intermediate level* (page 87) **OR** Exploring Your Neighborhood, *intermediate level* (page 85) **OR** Baby, Stroller, and You, *intermediate level* (page 117)
THURSDAY	Heart Healthy, *intermediate level* (page 105) **OR** No Joint Pain Necessary, *intermediate level* (page 108)
FRIDAY	Treadmill Walking, *intermediate level* (page 87) **OR** Now and Later, *intermediate level* (page 103) **OR** Hit the Beach! *intermediate level* (page 119)
SATURDAY	Strength-Training Workout, *intermediate level* (page 135)
SUNDAY	The Interval Workout, *intermediate level* (page 97) **OR** The Great Outdoors Workout #1, *advanced level* (page 99) **OR** Mall and Museum Walks, *intermediate level* (page 93)

Week #3

MONDAY	Treadmill Walking, *advanced level* (page 87) **OR** Heart Healthy, *advanced level* (page 105) **OR** Walking for the Fairway, *advanced level* (page 98)
TUESDAY	Strength-Training Workout, *advanced level* (page 135) **PLUS** Yoga and Pilates Routine (page 149)
WEDNESDAY	No Joint Pain Necessary, *advanced level* (page 108) **OR** Exploring Your Neighborhood, *advanced level* (page 85)
THURSDAY	Strength-Training Workout, *advanced level* (page 135) **PLUS** Yoga and Pilates Routine (page 149)
FRIDAY	Walking for Work, *advanced level* (page 90) **OR** Baby, Stroller, and You, *advanced level* (page 117)
SATURDAY	The Interval Workout, *advanced level* (page 97) **OR** The Great Outdoors Workout #2, *intermediate level* (page 101) **OR** Mall and Museum Walks, *advanced level* (page 93)
SUNDAY	Treadmill Walking, *advanced level* (page 87) **OR** Heart Healthy, *advanced level* (page 105) **OR** Walking for the Fairway, *advanced level* (page 98) **OR** Hit the Beach!, *advanced level* (page 119)

Week #4

MONDAY	The Interval Workout, *advanced level* (page 97) **OR** Now and Later, *advanced level* (page 103)
TUESDAY	Strength-Training Workout, *advanced level* (page 135) **PLUS** Yoga and Pilates Routine (page 149)
WEDNESDAY	Walking for the Fairway, *advanced level* (page 98) **OR** Treadmill Walking, *advanced level* (page 87) **OR** Mall and Museum Walks, *advanced level* (page 93)
THURSDAY	No Joint Pain Necessary, *advanced level* (page 108) **OR** Exploring Your Neighborhood, *advanced level* (page 85)
FRIDAY	Heart Healthy, *advanced level* (page 105) **OR** Baby, Stroller, and You, *intermediate level* (page 117)
SATURDAY	Strength-Training Workout, *advanced level* (page 135) **PLUS** Yoga and Pilates Routine (page 149)
SUNDAY	The Interval Workout, *advanced level* (page 97) **OR** Now and Later, *advanced level* (page 103) **OR** The Great Outdoors Workout #2, *intermediate level* (page 101)

Month #4 Workout Program

Complete the following monthly workout plan after finishing month #3. During this month, you'll be doing mostly advanced-level walking workouts 6 days a week. You'll also be completing my Strength-Training Workout 3 days a week, which means that some days you'll be doing both a walking workout and the Strength-Training Workout.

If your business or vacation plans take you away from home during this month, complete my Business and Vacation Travel workout on page 111, advanced level, instead of the suggested workout for that day. And if the day turns out to be cold and snowy, substitute the suggested workout with the Winter Wonderland workout, advanced level, on page 120.

Week #1

MONDAY	Treadmill Walking, *advanced level* (page 87) **OR** The Interval Workout, *advanced level* (page 97)
TUESDAY	Strength-Training Workout, *advanced level* (page 135) **PLUS** Yoga and Pilates Routine (page 149)
WEDNESDAY	No Joint Pain Necessary, *advanced level* (page 108) **OR** Walking for the Fairway, *advanced level* (page 98)
THURSDAY	Strength-Training Workout, *advanced level* (page 135) **PLUS** Treadmill Walking, *advanced level* (page 87) **OR** The Interval Workout, *advanced level* (page 97)
FRIDAY	Heart Healthy, *advanced level* (page 105) **OR** The Great Outdoors Workout #2, *advanced level* (page 101) **OR** Now and Later, *advanced level* (page 103)
SATURDAY	Strength-Training Workout, *advanced level* (page 135) **PLUS** The Interval Workout, *advanced level* (page 97) **OR** Hit the Beach! *advanced level* (page 119)
SUNDAY	Treadmill Walking, *advanced level* (page 87) **OR** Mall and Museum Walks, *advanced level* (page 93) **OR** Walking for Work, *advanced level* (page 90)

Week #2

MONDAY	Walking for Work, *advanced level* (page 90) **OR** No Joint Pain Necessary, *advanced level* (page 108) **OR** Walking for the Fairway, *advanced level* (page 98)
TUESDAY	Treadmill Walking, *advanced level* (page 87) **OR** Exploring Your Neighborhood, *advanced level* (page 85) **OR** Baby, Stroller, and You, *advanced level* (page 117)
WEDNESDAY	Strength-Training Workout, *advanced level* (page 135) **PLUS** Yoga and Pilates Routine (page 149)
THURSDAY	Heart Healthy, *advanced level* (page 105) **OR** The Great Outdoors Workout #2, *advanced level* (page 101) **OR** The Interval Workout, *advanced level* (page 97)
FRIDAY	Strength-Training Workout, *advanced level* (page 135) **PLUS** Treadmill Walking, *advanced level* (page 87) **OR** Now and Later, *advanced level* (page 103)
SATURDAY	The Great Outdoors Workout #1, *advanced level* (page 99) **OR** Mall and Museum Walks, *advanced level* (page 93)
SUNDAY	Strength-Training Workout, *advanced level* (page 135) **PLUS** The Interval Workout, *advanced level* (page 97) **OR** Hit the Beach! *advanced level* (page 119)

Week #3

MONDAY	Walking for the Fairway, *advanced level* (page 98) **OR** Treadmill Walking, *advanced level* (page 87)
TUESDAY	Strength-Training Workout, *advanced level* (page 135) **PLUS** Heart Healthy, *advanced level* (page 105) **OR** Now and Later, *advanced level* (page 103)
WEDNESDAY	No Joint Pain Necessary, *advanced level* (page 108) **OR** Exploring Your Neighborhood, *advanced level* (page 85)
THURSDAY	Strength-Training Workout, *advanced level* (page 135) **PLUS** Yoga and Pilates Routine (page 149)
FRIDAY	Walking for Work, *advanced level* (page 90) **OR** Baby, Stroller, and You, *advanced level* (page 117) **OR** The Great Outdoors Workout #2, *advanced level* (page 101)
SATURDAY	Strength-Training Workout, *advanced level* (page 135) **PLUS** The Interval Workout, *advanced level* (page 97) **OR** Hit the Beach! *advanced level* (page 119)
SUNDAY	Walking for the Fairway, *advanced level* (page 98) **OR** Treadmill Walking, *advanced level* (page 87) **OR** Mall and Museum Walks, *advanced level* (page 93)

Week #4

MONDAY	Strength-Training Workout, *advanced level* (page 135) **PLUS** Interval Workout, *advanced level* (page 97) **OR** Heart Healthy, *advanced level* (page 105)
TUESDAY	Walking for the Fairway, *advanced level* (page 98) **OR** Baby, Stroller, and You, *advanced level* (page 117) **OR** No Joint Pain Necessary, *advanced level* (page 108)
WEDNESDAY	Strength-Training Workout, *advanced level* (page 135) **PLUS** Walking for Work, *advanced level* (page 90) **OR** Treadmill Walking, *advanced level* (page 87)
THURSDAY	Heart Healthy, *advanced level* (page 105) **OR** The Interval Workout, *advanced level* (page 97) **OR** Now and Later, *advanced level* (page 103)
FRIDAY	Strength-Training Workout, *advanced level* (page 135) **PLUS** Yoga and Pilates Routine (page 149)
SATURDAY	Now and Later, *advanced level* (page 103) **OR** Treadmill Walking, *advanced level* (page 87) **OR** Hit the Beach! *advanced level* (page 119)
SUNDAY	Mall and Museum Walks, *advanced level* (page 93) **OR** The Interval Workout, *advanced level* (page 97) **OR** The Great Outdoors Workout #2, *advanced level* (page 101)

The Warm-Weather Workout Program

I'm a firm believer in fitting your exercise plan to your lifestyle, not the other way around. That's why I've created the following Warm-Weather Workout Program. If you live in an area where the four seasons are distinct, you're probably eager to get outdoors after a long winter. The following program gives you the chance to take advantage of the beautiful weather. It's jam-packed with workouts that get you outside, whether it's simply exploring the blossoming flowers and trees as you walk in your neighborhood, heading to the beach for a workout, gearing up to hit the links, or preparing for your summer camping trip. And on rainy days or days when the weather is a little *too* warm, you'll have the option of doing your workout indoors—either on a treadmill or in an air-conditioned mall or museum. This program is also great if you're fortunate enough to live where the weather conditions are mild all year long, such as in the southern United States.

Note: Complete the beginner, intermediate, or advanced levels of each workout below depending on your fitness level. If you choose to substitute this program as the first month of your exercise program, complete all workouts at the beginner level. If you've already completed either the Month #1 or Month #2 Workout Program or have already been working out consistently for an hour or more at least three times a week, complete this program at the intermediate level. Finally, if you've completed the Month #3 or Month #4 Workout Program, complete this program at the advanced level.

Note: If you're doing the advanced-level workouts, be sure to add in the optional Yoga and Pilates Routine on the days you do your strength-training workouts. (You will also be doing the Yoga and Pilates Routine after you complete each advanced-level walking workout.)

Week #1

MONDAY	Exploring Your Neighborhood (page 85) **OR** Walking for Work (page 90) **OR** Hit the Beach! (page 119)
TUESDAY	Strength-Training Workout (page 135) **PLUS** Yoga and Pilates Routine, optional (page 149)
WEDNESDAY	Walking for the Fairway (page 98) **OR** Interval Workout (page 97)
THURSDAY	Strength-Training Workout (page 135) **PLUS** Yoga and Pilates Routine, optional (page 149)
FRIDAY	Now and Later (page 103) **OR** Heart Healthy (page 105)
SATURDAY	Mall and Museum Walks (page 93) **OR** The Great Outdoors Workout #1 (page 99)
SUNDAY	Exploring Your Neighborhood (page 85) **OR** Walking for Work (page 90) **OR** Hit the Beach! (page 119)

Week #2

MONDAY	Hit the Beach! (page 119) **OR** No Joint Pain Necessary (page 108) **OR** Walking for Work (page 90)
TUESDAY	Strength-Training Workout (page 135) **PLUS** Yoga and Pilates Routine, optional (page 149)
WEDNESDAY	Exploring Your Neighborhood (page 85) **OR** Mall and Museum Walks (page 93)
THURSDAY	The Great Outdoors Workout #1 (page 99) **OR** Heart Healthy (page 105)
FRIDAY	Now and Later (page 103) **OR** Baby, Stroller, and You (page 117) **OR** Treadmill Walking (page 87)
SATURDAY	Strength-Training Workout (page 135) **PLUS** Yoga and Pilates Routine, optional (page 149)
SUNDAY	Hit the Beach! (page 119) **OR** No Joint Pain Necessary (page 108) **OR** Walking for Work (page 90)

Week #3

MONDAY	Hit the Beach! (page 119) **OR** Heart Healthy (page 105) **OR** Treadmill Walking (page 87)
TUESDAY	Strength-Training Workout (page 135) **PLUS** Yoga and Pilates Routine, optional (page 149)
WEDNESDAY	Exploring Your Neighborhood (page 85) **OR** No Joint Pain Necessary (page 108)
THURSDAY	Strength-Training Workout (page 135) **PLUS** Yoga and Pilates Routine, optional (page 149)
FRIDAY	Walking for Work (page 90) **OR** The Great Outdoors, Workout #2 (page 101)
SATURDAY	The Interval Workout (page 97) **OR** Mall and Museum Walks (page 93)
SUNDAY	Hit the Beach! (page 119) **OR** Heart Healthy (page 105) **OR** Treadmill Walking (page 87)

Week #4

MONDAY	The Great Outdoors Workout #2 (page 101) **OR** Walking for the Fairway (page 98) **OR** The Interval Workout (page 97)
TUESDAY	Strength-Training Workout (page 135) **PLUS** Yoga and Pilates Routine, optional (page 149)
WEDNESDAY	Now and Later (page 103) **OR** Treadmill Walking (page 87) **OR** No Joint Pain Necessary (page 108)
THURSDAY	Exploring Your Neighborhood (page 85) **OR** Mall and Museum Walks (page 93)
FRIDAY	Heart Healthy (page 105) **OR** Baby, Stroller, and You (page 117)
SATURDAY	Strength-Training Workout (page 135) **PLUS** Yoga and Pilates Routine, optional (page 149)
SUNDAY	The Great Outdoors Workout #2 (page 101) **OR** Walking for the Fairway (page 98) **OR** The Interval Workout (page 97)

The Cold-Weather Workout Program

When it's chilly outside and the wind is whistling around the walls of your house, it can be hard to work up the motivation to get outdoors and exercise. That's why I've created the following Cold-Weather Workout Program. This program gives you plenty of indoor options so that you can get a safe, effective workout even when, as the song says, "the weather outside is frightful." And for those days when the thermometer does creep upward, you'll have the chance to try out my Winter Wonderland workout. Finally, because exercising in cold weather can require creativity, this program also leans heavily on the Now and Later workout, which allows you to get your workout for the day in short bursts, so that you're not outside for more than a few minutes at a time. Plus, it's ideal for fitting in a 10- or 15-minute walk over your lunch hour, when the sun is shining and the wind doesn't feel quite so cold. (This is especially great when Daylight Savings Time means that it's already dark when you get home from work.)

Note: Complete the beginner, intermediate, or advanced levels of each workout below depending on your fitness level. If you choose to substitute this program as the first month of your exercise program, complete all workouts at the beginner level. If you've already completed either the Month #1 or Month #2 Workout Program or have already been working out consistently for an hour or more at least three times a week, complete this program at the *intermediate level*. Finally, if you've completed the Month #3 or Month #4 Workout Program, complete this program at the advanced level.

Note: If you're doing the advanced-level workouts, be sure to add in the optional Yoga and Pilates Routine on the days you do your strength-training workouts. (You will also be doing the Yoga and Pilates Routine after you complete each advanced-level walking workout.)

Week #1

MONDAY	Treadmill Walking (page 87) **OR** Mall and Museum Walks (page 93)
TUESDAY	Strength-Training Workout (page 135) **PLUS** Yoga and Pilates Routine, optional (page 149)
WEDNESDAY	Winter Wonderland Workout (page 120) **OR** Now and Later (page 103)
THURSDAY	Strength-Training Workout (page 135) **PLUS** Yoga and Pilates Routine, optional (page 149)
FRIDAY	Now and Later (page 103) **OR** Heart Healthy (page 105)
SATURDAY	Mall and Museum Walks (page 93) **OR** Walking for Work (page 90)
SUNDAY	Treadmill Walking (page 87) **OR** Mall and Museum Walks (page 93)

Week #2

MONDAY	Now and Later (page 103) **OR** Winter Wonderland (page 120)
TUESDAY	Strength-Training Workout (page 135) **PLUS** Yoga and Pilates Routine, optional (page 149)
WEDNESDAY	Treadmill Walking (page 87) **OR** Exploring Your Neighborhood (page 85)
THURSDAY	Heart Healthy (page 105) **OR** No Joint Pain Necessary (page 108)
FRIDAY	Treadmill Walking (page 87) **OR** Now and Later (page 103)
SATURDAY	Strength-Training Workout (page 135) **PLUS** Yoga and Pilates Routine, optional (page 149)
SUNDAY	Mall and Museum Walks (page 93) **OR** Winter Wonderland (page 120)

Week #3

MONDAY	Treadmill Walking (page 87) **OR** Heart Healthy (page 105) **OR** Now and Later (page 103)
TUESDAY	Strength-Training Workout (page 135) **PLUS** Yoga and Pilates Routine, optional (page 149)
WEDNESDAY	Mall and Museum Walks (page 93) **OR** Winter Wonderland (page 120)
THURSDAY	Strength-Training Workout (page 135) **PLUS** Yoga and Pilates Routine, optional (page 149)
FRIDAY	Mall and Museum Walks (page 93) **OR** Walking for Work (page 90)
SATURDAY	Now and Later (page 103) **OR** Winter Wonderland (page 120)
SUNDAY	Treadmill Walking (page 87) **OR** Heart Healthy (page 105) **OR** Mall and Museum Walks (page 93)

Week #4

MONDAY	Now and Later (page 103) **OR** Winter Wonderland (page 120)
TUESDAY	Strength-Training Workout (page 135) **PLUS** Yoga and Pilates Routine, optional (page 149)
WEDNESDAY	Treadmill Walking (page 87) **OR** Exploring Your Neighborhood (page 85)
THURSDAY	Mall and Museum Walks (page 93) **OR** Walking for Work (page 90)
FRIDAY	Treadmill Walking (page 87) **OR** Now and Later (page 103)
SATURDAY	Strength-Training Workout (page 135) **PLUS** Yoga and Pilates Routine, optional (page 149)
SUNDAY	Mall and Museum Walks (page 93) **OR** Winter Wonderland (page 120)

Extending the Program

If you've completed my 4-month workout program, you've no doubt shed significant pounds and toned and strengthened your body in the process. I'll bet you look
and feel great. Congratulations! Give yourself a pat on the back; you deserve it!

Now that you've seen what a difference an active lifestyle can make, keep that
momentum going! Go back to the monthly programs and try mixing them up in
new combinations. Use your Walking Logs to recall which workouts you completed
each day, then try out one of the other options for that day. The possibilities are
endless, and the only thing you have to lose is more weight!

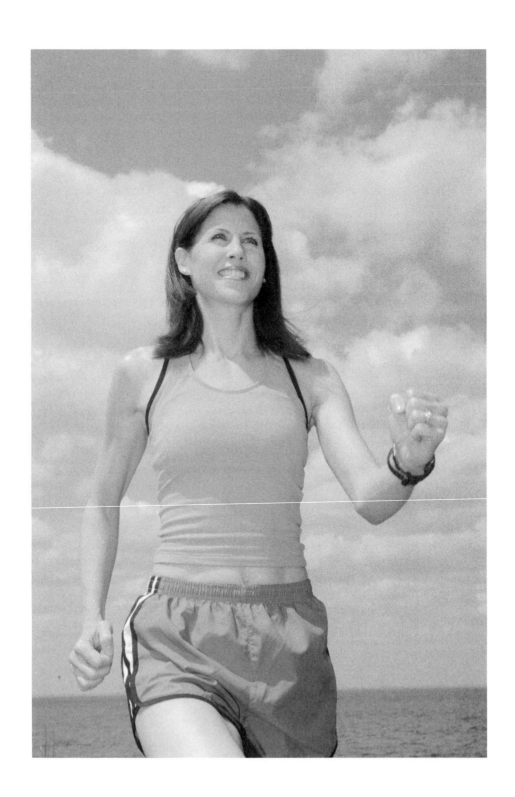

CHAPTER FIVE
The Walking Workouts

I N THIS CHAPTER, YOU'LL DISCOVER my 16 walking workouts. There's so much here from which to choose, everything from walks in malls to walks on trails, in stadiums, and at the beach. For each workout, I've explained its benefits and then detailed exactly how to do the workout. For each workout, I offer a plan for beginners and then variations for intermediate and advanced walkers. Unless you've been working out consistently for an hour or more at least three times a week, start with the beginner level of each workout and work your way up to the more advanced levels, following my 4-Month Program (see page 55).

Exploring Your Neighborhood

This basic workout is perfect when you want a no-frills routine that doesn't require any advance planning, such as getting yourself to the gym. Our initial goal for this program is to explore our surroundings to see what different types of routes we can take in the future, and then to establish our favorites. These will become tried-and-true workouts that we can rely on whenever we don't want to have to put a lot of mental energy into choosing a workout.

- To prepare your heart, lungs, and muscles for exercise, ease in with a light warm-up of walking for 10 minutes at an easy pace.
- Next, complete the following two moves, which will warm up and stretch your muscles, preparing them for the workout ahead:
  Knee-to-Chest Warm-Up: While standing erect, lift one leg off the ground. Grasp it with both hands above or below the knee, pulling your leg up to your chest. Hold for 30 seconds. Alternate with the other leg and repeat 2 times.

Side-to-Side Twist: With your arms hanging comfortably at your sides, twist your upper body and arms to both sides while lightly swinging your arms around your body. Allow your lower body to follow the movement with a concurrent weight transfer. Complete 8 to 10 rotations, holding each for 10 seconds.

- You're now ready to begin your fitness walk! Start walking in your neighborhood at a light pace of approximately 3 to 4 mph. Our goal today is to walk for 20 minutes, roughly 1 to 1.5 miles. After you complete your 20-minute walk, use your car to measure the distance that you completed. Or, if you'd prefer, you can use your pedometer to estimate the distance. Once you've completed this workout a number of times, you'll have a few different routes at various distances.

    Key points to remember: Think about your posture as you walk. Be sure to look forward, not down, and to keep your upper body and spine in a neutral position. The essence of good posture is a natural skeletal balance maintained by muscles strong enough to hold everything in place. It's almost impossible to have good posture and not be fit. Maintaining good posture will keep you from tiring early in your upper body before you can complete your exercise.

    As you walk, relax your shoulders, breathe naturally, and enjoy! You'll burn approximately 150 calories during this exercise.

- After you've completed your 20-minute fitness walk, cool down by walking for 5 minutes at one-half to one-quarter of your previous pace.
- Finally, stretch out the muscles you've just worked by completing the Post-Workout Stretching Routine on page 129.

    Intermediate Level: Increase the duration of your fitness walk to 45 minutes. You'll burn approximately 400 calories during this walk. Be sure to warm up your muscles first with a slower-paced 10-minute walk and cool down for 5 minutes afterward. Finish by completing the Post-Workout Stretching Routine on page 129.

    Advanced Level: Complete the Intermediate-Level workout explained above, including the 5-minute cooldown walk. Next, complete the Yoga and Pilates Routine on page 149. (You want your muscles to be warm for the Yoga and Pilates routine, so cool down after your walking workout, but don't sit down.) Finish with the Post-Workout Stretching Routine on page 129.

Treadmill Walking

When the weather forces you indoors or you're simply not in the mood for an out-door workout, treadmills (whether at a gym or a home version in your basement) offer a great alternative. In fact, in a study reported in the *Journal of the American Medical Association,* treadmills were found to be the best means of energy expenditure and aerobic exercise when compared to a cross-country skier, a rowing machine, a stair climber, and a stationary bike. The study showed that both walking and running on a treadmill at moderate to intense levels induced significantly higher rates of energy expenditure and raised heart rate substantially over other forms of indoor exercise.

What's more, because the treadmill surface is softer than pavement, walking on it is a little easier on our joints. So if you suffer from knee pain or soreness, opt for treadmill workouts frequently.

- To prepare your heart, lungs, and muscles for exercise, ease in with a light warm-up of walking on your treadmill for 10 minutes at an easy pace, with no grade set.

  Minutes 1 to 5: Once you've completed your warm-up, it's time to start your fitness walk. For the first 5 minutes of your fitness walk, set the speed to 3 mph and the incline, or grade, at 2 degrees. This setting not only increases the intensity of the exercise but allows the foot to land in a more efficient manner. It forces the heel, rather than the mid- or fore-foot, to strike upon reaching the surface; mid- or forefoot strikes can increase your chances for developing shin splints. (Shin splints occur when the muscles on the back of the lower legs become overdeveloped and lose flexibility. In addition to setting a small grade on the treadmill, be sure to stretch after every exercise session to further prevent shin splints. Doing exercises to strengthen the front side of the lower leg, such as the Calf Stretch on Step described on page 130, will also reduce your chance of shin splints.) Plus, some studies suggest that when you walk indoors, you expend about 5 percent fewer calories because you're not fighting against the wind resistance of outdoor walking. By setting your treadmill at an incline of 2 degrees, you can easily make up for this difference. For the rest of your walk, follow this guide.

  Minutes 6 to 10: Set the speed to 3.7 mph and raise the incline to 3 degrees.

  Minutes 11 to 20: Set the speed to 3.9 mph and keep the incline at 3 degrees.

What to Look For When Buying a Home Treadmill

According to the Sporting Goods Manufacturers Association, 11.6 million Americans worked out on treadmills regularly in 2003. And a lot of those folks worked out on treadmills in their homes.

If you simply don't have the space or desire for a home treadmill, you can easily complete my Treadmill Walking workout on a treadmill at your local gym. But if you enjoy working out on a treadmill and think having one at home would motivate you to work out more frequently, purchasing one will be a great investment. There are many different brands of treadmills on the market, and it seems like they're sold almost everywhere. Before you part with your hard-earned money, consider the tips below.

If you can afford it, choose motorized over manual. Your first decision will be to decide if you want a motorized or a manual treadmill. Unfortunately, there are many drawbacks to manual versions: They're difficult to get moving without using an extreme incline, and once you are moving, you have no other options. You can't change the incline. Although they cost less, they are usually less sturdy. With motorized treadmills, you can adjust the speed and choose from various workout program options that will give you a varied workout. This can push you to work harder. Plus, the constantly moving belt of a motorized treadmill can motivate you to simply keep going.

Consider the treadmill's features and benefits. Take the time to acquaint yourself with the specific features of any treadmill you're considering purchasing. Here are a few things, in particular, to consider.

- Most people find the use of electronic programming on motorized treadmills very useful. This is the button that automatically increases or decreases your workout intensity and grade—the way walking up and down real hills does outdoors.

- The second most important feature on a treadmill is ample stability and cushioning. This concern was laid to rest for me when I purchased my first treadmill, which was made by the top-notch fitness equipment manufacturer True. This company uses special-grade shock-absorbing treads that make their treadmills most impact-friendly. I really believe its soft cushion saved my neck and back.

- Next, be sure the treadmill you're considering has a strong frame. And for safety reasons, you want a treadmill with a large walking belt so you don't have to worry about accidentally stepping off of it. You also want to make sure that the hand rails are easy to grip and sturdy to the touch.

- Another concern for many people is the loudness of the treadmill's motor. For example, I need a treadmill with a quiet motor because I like to walk when my children are napping; a noisy machine would wake the kids and blow my workout. Also, if you plan to watch TV, listen to music, or turn on that baby monitor during your workout, you'll need to hear those noises over the treadmill motor.

Never purchase a treadmill without trying it out first. How else will you know how the treadmill will feel as you work out on it? Be sure to wear your walking shoes and comfortable clothes when you test the treadmills you're considering. Carefully consider the features and benefits we just discussed.

Check the warranty. Better warranties offer lifetime coverage on the frame, at least 3 years on the motor, and 1-year labor coverage.

Consider the treadmill's optional features. For example, a pulse monitor is a useful feature you'll be glad to have. A place for your water bottle and a magazine or book rack are nice features as well.

Read the review. For more information on how the treadmill you're considering stacks up against the competition, check out www.TtreadmillDdoctor.com, which is a great online source for treadmill reviews.

Minutes 21 to 25: Set the speed to 4.1 mph and raise the incline to 5 degrees.

Minutes 26 to 30: Slow the speed to 3.7 mph and lower the incline to 1 degree.

- Congratulations, you've finished your fitness work on the treadmill! Next, cool down by walking on the treadmill (set at 0 grade) for 5 minutes at one-half to one-quarter of your previous pace.

- After your treadmill workout, complete the following stretch, which will stretch out your calves and hopefully keep those shin splints away forever.

Calf Stretch: Find a stair and step up on it with both feet. Hang your heels off the back of the stair. If needed, you can balance your upper body by holding onto a railing or wall. Stretch each leg by alternately lowering the heel below the level of the stair. Keep your knee on the extended leg soft, not locked. Hold each stretch for 20 to 30 seconds. Do 5 reps on each leg, being careful not to bounce.

- Finally, stretch out the rest of your body by completing the Post-Workout Stretching Routine on page 129.

Intermediate Level: After completing a warm-up of 10 minutes at a slower pace, complete the following 35-minute workout.

Minutes 1 to 5: Same as above

Minutes 6 to 10: Same as above

Minutes 11 to 20: Set the speed to 3.9 mph, but raise the incline to 7 degrees.

Minutes 21 to 35: Set the speed to 4.1 mph and increase the incline to 10 degrees.

- Finally, cool down by walking on the treadmill (set at 0 grade) for 5 minutes at one-half to one-quarter of your previous pace.

- After your treadmill workout, complete the calf stretch, as described above. Finish with the Post-Workout Stretching Routine on page 129.

Advanced Level: Complete the Intermediate Level workout explained above. After completing the calf stretch, do the Yoga and Pilates Routine found on page 149. Finish with the Post-Workout Stretching Routine on page 129.

Walking for Work

Climbing up flights of stairs, getting into and out of our cars, running to catch the bus—each day, we depend on our muscles, and especially the muscles in our legs, to get us through the demands of our busy schedules. And when those muscles aren't toned, we can end up feeling tired, weak, worn out—or even injured. The following workout will not only help you shed pounds but will also help strengthen the muscles you need to complete your daily work and move easily through your busy day. And when you're able to move through your day more easily, you'll be more likely to be more active *between* your workouts—resulting in an even greater calorie burn, stronger muscles, and a more agile you.

- To prepare your heart, lungs, and muscles for exercise, ease in with a light warm-up of walking for 10 minutes at an easy pace.

• Next, find a sturdy staircase or a makeshift step about 8 inches tall that will support your body weight to complete the following exercise.

> **Step-Up:** Step up onto the stair or box leading with your right foot and follow the right with the left until both feet have ascended together. (As you step up, lead with your heel and be sure to keep your knees in line with your toes on top of the step.) Step down with the right and then the left foot. That's 1 repetition. Complete this move for 20 repetitions. Then do another 20 reps, this time leading with your left foot.
>
> *Note:* The Reebok steps work really well for this move. To purchase, visit a sporting goods store near you.

• You're now ready to begin the walking portion of the workout. Today, we're going to add a strength-training exercise into our walking routine. Before setting out, be sure to grab a watch or stopwatch. Our goal today is to walk for 25 minutes at 3 to 4 mph. Every 2 minutes, we'll stop walking and perform 20 squats, which are excellent for strengthening the quadriceps, hamstrings, and gluteals.

> **Squat:** To perform a squat correctly, stand with your feet slightly wider than shoulder-width apart, bearing the majority of the weight on your heels. Next sit your hips backward away from your body, while keeping your eyes and chin up at a 45-degree angle relative to the ground. With your arms out in front of you, begin to perform a sitting move until your knees have reached an angle of about 90 degrees, but never more than that. Keep your back in a neutral position, never arched. One repetition should take about 5 seconds (2 seconds descending, 1 second pause, and 2 seconds ascending). Each set of 20 reps should take approximately 1½ minutes. After completing 20 reps, begin walking again at the same pace. Keep in mind, every 2 minutes of walking should be followed by a 1½-minute squat set.

• After you've completed your 25-minute fitness walk with 2-minute splits, cool down by walking for 5 minutes at one-half to one-quarter of your previous pace.

• Finally, stretch out the muscles you've just worked by completing the Post-Workout Stretching Routine on page 129.

> *Intermediate Level:* After warming up your muscles first with a slower-paced 10-minute walk, complete 45 minutes at a brisk walking pace of 4 to 5 mph, including the 2-minute splits with squats of 30 repetitions

Self-Healing and Injury Relief

In terms of injury risk, walking is one of the safest exercise options you can choose. Still, walkers may occasionally experience a minor overuse injury, typically when they're first beginning an intense walking program. To treat these injuries—and prevent them in the future—I recommend a three-step approach: Stretch, ice, and massage.

Stretch: Properly stretching out your muscles will go a long way toward preventing pain and injury. In fact, one of the most common overuse injuries, shin splints, is best prevented by stretching. (See Calf Stretch on Step on page 130.) Shin splints are caused by an overdevelopment or overuse of the calf muscles. If you don't stretch out your calf muscles after working out, they can become shorter and shorter over time. Eventually the standard distance they're designed to travel is also shortened, but the tendons holding them to the bony structures in your body don't give as easily, so they strain and ache, and often become inflamed.

Another common complaint among new walkers is lower-back pain. Often, this is associated with referral pain caused by a lack of flexibility in the legs. The hamstrings, which run behind your thighs and knees, are often the most overlooked, improperly stretched muscles in the body. The hamstrings are often much weaker than the larger-by-design quadriceps, and many overuse injuries are caused by this imbalance in strength and flexibility. This imbalanced equation results in combative forces on your hips and lower back.

Any time there is an imbalance somewhere in the body, your body will naturally attempt to correct or accommodate it by adjusting posture or limiting range of motion to minimize injury. As these subtle differences occur and cause low levels of pain, you might feel as though you can "walk through it" and it will just go away. In most cases, this doesn't happen. Instead, the condition continues and intensifies. If you're experiencing lower-back pain, try the Seated Hamstring Stretch on page 130.

Note: If stretching your lower body doesn't help to relieve your pain and discomfort, visit a sports medicine doctor, podiatrist, or physical therapist. Either of these professionals can test your gait pattern, strength, and flexibility and test for possible injuries. With this information, he or she can help you to develop a plan of action that will get you back on the path to pain-free exercise.

Ice: In addition to stretching, optimal management of an acute injury can best be remembered by the acronym RICE.

Rest: Minimize movement of the injured body part.

Ice: Wrap ice in a towel and apply it for 20 minutes every 2 hours for the first 48 hours. Keep in mind, however, that some people with circulatory problems as well as children and the elderly may be more sensitive to cold and you should adjust your treatment accordingly.

Compression: Apply a light pressure wrap to help minimize bleeding and swelling.

Elevation: Raise the injured body part to allow fluids to drain from the affected area, which will reduce the pressure from blood and tissue swelling.

Use heat to treat stiff muscles and joints, but do not use it in the first days after an injury, because it may increase blood flow and worsen swelling. Apply it for 15 to 20 minutes, but use caution as heat packs that are too hot or left in place for too long may cause burns.

Massage: This is the final component to self-healing and injury prevention for active individuals. If you don't want to hire a massage therapist, go out and buy a self-massaging tool. There are hundreds of items on the market; test out a few different ones at your local athletic store to see which one works best for you. Massage helps realign well-worked muscle fiber strains, and it also helps to flush out the toxins produced during exercise. It can return the muscle to its relaxed length, too.

instead of 20. Cool down with a slower-paced walk for 5 minutes. End with the Post-Workout Stretching Routine on page 129.

Advanced Level: Complete the Intermediate-Level workout explained above. After your 5-minute cooldown, complete the Yoga and Pilates Routine on page 149. Finish with the Post-Workout Stretching Routine on page 129.

Mall and Museum Walks

Finally, there's a workout that gives you permission to "shop till you drop"! Unlike other trips to the mall, though, the following workout won't cost you a dime; in fact, you'll be burning tons of calories while your cash burns a hole in your pocket!

Have you ever spent an afternoon at the mall or exploring a local museum, art gallery, or aquarium? Chances are the time flew by as you walked from store to store or exhibit to exhibit. And I'd be willing to bet that when you finally got back home, you felt pretty tired. That's because as you shop or visit a museum, you're logging hundreds of steps (often without even thinking about it)—especially if your adventure takes you through a large, multi-level shopping mall or museum.

Today, we're going to harness that energy expenditure and boost it even further for maximum calorie-burning potential. The following workout is perfect for rainy or snowy days, evenings when you don't feel safe walking outdoors, or days when you just can't motivate yourself to do a treadmill workout. And don't forget—malls, museums, and other public buildings are air-conditioned, so they're the perfect workout spot for hot, humid days. And if you have allergies, malls and museums—with their dry, filtered air—can offer a welcome respite from the pollen and dust you'd encounter outdoors. But even if the weather is gorgeous, mixing up your workout plan with a mall or museum workout can be a great motivational tool. Let's face it: Going to a mall or museum is just plain fun! You'll get to see lots of people and do a little (fast-paced!) window-shopping or (if your walk takes you to a museum or art gallery) perhaps pick up a little culture along the way!

Be creative when looking for places to do this workout. Your local mall is a great option, and some malls open early just for mall walkers. If yours doesn't, you might try talking with the mall manager to see if arrangements could be made to allow early hours for mall walkers. Of course, doing your walks during off-hours, such as the early morning or over lunch on weekdays, will allow you to bypass most of the crowds. If you live in a city, you could also try a museum, large public library, or other large building open to the public. And if you work in a large, multi-level office building, try this workout there.

Part of the beauty of malls, museums, and other large public buildings is that they typically have one of the greatest pieces of exercise equipment—stairs! Taking the stairs increases your metabolic rate 6 to 8 times while you're stepping. At rest, your body burns an average of 3 to 5 calories per minute, and as soon as you begin walking, that number increases by 2.5 times. But the real boost comes when you take the stairs. As soon as you do, that number jumps up to 8 times your resting metabolic rate, meaning that you burn a whopping 25 to 40 calories every minute you spend walking up those stairs. Wow!

To get in on the fun, try out the following walking workout, which will allow you to burn up to 500 calories—that's equivalent to running 5 miles. And when you add in the strength-training work, you'll burn additional calories all day long. Remember: One pound of lean muscle mass requires 35 calories every day just to maintain itself. On the other hand, 1 pound of fat tissue requires only 2 to 3 calories per day. So the more muscle we have, the more calories we burn, even at rest. Plus, a pound of muscle takes up less space than a pound of fat, so you can get into smaller jeans without actually losing weight.

- To prepare your muscles for exercise, begin with a light warm-up of walking for 10 minutes through the mall, museum, art gallery, or aquarium at an easy pace.
- Next, find a little-used hallway with a bench to do the following targeted strength-training moves.

    Walking Lunge: Take a large step forward, while maintaining a tall, upright upper body. Strike the lead foot, keeping the weight on the heel and midfoot. Next, drop down by bending your back knee. Don't let your back knee touch the floor. Pause at the bottom, and then stand back up by lifting your back leg as you travel down the hallway or sidewalk. Your hands and arms can be by your side, or wherever you feel balanced, but don't place them on your legs for assistance. Complete 3 sets of 10 walking lunges on each leg.

    Bench Dip: First, find a deserted bench. Face away from it and place your hands flat on the seat, extending your feet a couple of feet in front of you. This is easier when you keep your weight in your heels. Keeping your elbows close to your sides, slowly lower yourself until your upper arms are parallel to the floor. Slowly push back up and repeat. Complete 3 sets of 10 to 12 dips each.

Wall or Bench Push-Up: Stand about 3 feet in front of a wall, with your feet shoulder-width apart. Place your hands at shoulder-height on the wall; they should be slightly more than shoulder-width apart. Bend your arms and slowly lower yourself toward the wall, keeping your body straight, like a plank. Concentrate on contracting your abdominal muscles and be careful not to allow your head to bend forward or backward. Try to get as close to the wall as possible, hold for a count of 2, and then slowly push away.

Alternately, you can do these push-ups using a bench. (Place your hands shoulder-width apart on the bench.) However, when doing push-ups on a bench, pay particular attention to keeping your abs in and not arching your back. Complete 3 sets of 10 to 12 push-ups each.

- Next comes your fitness walk. Our goal for today is to walk for an hour, dividing up that time with some calorie-burning stairwork. Every 10 minutes, I want you to find a staircase and go up and down it for 5 minutes. Once the 5 minutes are up, continue walking. When the hour is complete, you'll have done 20 minutes of stairwork—truly a great accomplishment!

- Next, cool down by walking for 5 minutes at one-half to one-quarter of your previous pace.

- Finally, stretch out the muscles you've just worked by completing the Post-Workout Stretching Routine on page 129.

Intermediate Level: Complete the workout as described above, but increase the number of reps for each of the strength-training moves, as follows:

Walking Lunge: Complete 3 sets of 15 lunges on each leg.

Bench Dip: Complete 3 sets of 15 to 20 dips each.

Wall or Bench Push-Up: Complete 3 sets of 15 to 20 push-ups each.

After your 1-hour fitness walk with stair-climbing intervals, don't forget to end with a 5-minute cooldown walk at one-half to one-quarter of your previous pace. Then finish up with the Post-Workout Stretching Routine on page 129.

Advanced Level: Complete the Intermediate-Level workout explained above. After your 5-minute cooldown, complete the Yoga and Pilates Routine on page 149. Finish with the Post-Workout Stretching Routine on page 129.

The Interval Workout

We've already established that walking burns 2.5 times the number of calories per minute than when we're at rest. As you might imagine, running burns even more. Just like taking the stairs, a light running pace burns up to 8 times the number of calories per minute than when we're at rest. Remember the biggest difference between walking and running is flight, meaning there is a moment with each stride that both feet are airborne.

Beginning a walking/running program is a smart way to increase the intensity of your workouts, without increasing the risk of injury. So on days when you're ready for a challenge, try the following workout.

- To prepare your muscles for exercise, begin with a light warm-up of walking for 10 minutes at an easy pace.
- Next, walk for 10 minutes at a moderate pace (2.5 to 3.5) mph, about as fast as you would cross the street at a cross walk...not so fast that you might look like you're in a hurry, but fast enough so that you're on the other side before the light turns green! This moderately paced walk will prepare your muscles and joints for a light run.
- Now run for 3 minutes at a comfortable pace. When the 3 minutes are up, walk for 5 minutes. Repeat 3 times.

    Note: Unlike some of the other workouts in this book, you'll want to increase the difficulty of this workout each time you do it. Refer to the Intermediate-Level instructions below to learn how to do this.

- Next, cool down by walking for 5 minutes at one-half to one-quarter of your previous walking pace.
- Finally, stretch out the muscles you've just worked by completing the Post-Workout Stretching Routine on page 129.

    Intermediate Level: To increase the intensity of this workout, increase the amount of time you run by 1 minute every time you try this routine, until you can complete 10-minute running intervals. Afterward, don't forget to cool down with a 5-minute walk at one-half to one-quarter of your previous walking pace. Finish by completing the Post-Workout Stretching Routine on page 129.

Advanced Level: Complete the Intermediate-Level workout explained above. After your 5-minute cooldown, complete the Yoga and Pilates Routine on page 149. Finish with the Post-Workout Stretching Routine on page 129.

Walking for the Fairway

In recent years, golf has become increasingly popular as men and women of all ages discover (or rediscover) the joys of the game. It's a great way to get some exercise, some fresh air, and spark that competitive drive. And, of course, if your colleagues are golfers, taking up the game can even be good for your career. The following workout will not only help you to walk the course with ease, but it also includes a few exercises to improve your game—and your health.

- To prepare your heart, lungs, and muscles for exercise, ease in with a light warm-up of walking for 10 minutes at an easy pace.
- Next, complete the following exercises, which are great for both your walking workout and your golf game.

  Knee-to-Chest Warm-Up: While standing erect, lift one leg off the ground. Grasp it with both hands above or below the knee, pulling your leg up to your chest. Hold for 5 seconds. Repeat with the other leg. Do 10 to 15 repetitions with each leg.

  Side Step: Take a large step to each side, bending your knees (but not as far as you would when doing a squat) and moving your body laterally and sitting your hips back behind you. Complete 20 repetitions to each side.

  Golf Club Stretch: Holding a golf club across your chest, cross both arms and rotate your upper body as if you were taking a swing. Back-swing, pause, and downswing to finish. Repeat for 20 reps. A proper shoulder turn will allow your torso to warm up and prepare you for the course.

- Our goal today is to walk for 1 hour. During a round of golf, we can spend nearly twice that long actually walking down the fairways. We'll also be adding some lunges to our walking workout. Be sure to wear a pedometer, watch, or stopwatch. Begin walking at a fairly quick pace, preferably 5 mph.

- For the first 30 minutes of your 1-hour walk, every 3 minutes, stop and complete the following exercise for 1 minute.

   Walking Lunge: Take a large step forward, while maintaining a tall, upright upper body. Strike the lead foot, keeping the weight on the heel and mid-foot. Next, drop down by bending your back knee. Don't let your back knee touch the ground because this allows the muscles to rest, and I don't want you to rest just yet. Continue with the other foot, alternating at a comfortable pace.

- For the second 30 minutes of your 1-hour walk, every 3 minutes, stop and complete 10 reps per side of the following exercise.

   Walking Lunge with Rotation: As you reach the bottom of the lunge, reach your arms out in front of you and rotate your upper body to the side of your body that has the forward leg on the ground. Rotate back to center, stand up, and complete the same on the opposing side.

- After completing your 1-hour fitness walk, cool down by walking for 5 minutes at one-half to one-quarter of your previous pace.

- Finally, stretch out the muscles you've just worked by completing the Post-Workout Stretching Routine on page 129.

   Intermediate Level: Begin by warming up your muscles with a slower-paced 10-minute walk. Then complete the fitness walk as described above, but double the repetitions of each additional exercise. Cool down with a slower-paced walk for 5 minutes. End by completing the Post-Workout Stretching Routine on page 129.

   Advanced Level: Complete the Intermediate-Level workout explained above. After your 5-minute cooldown, complete the Yoga and Pilates Routine on page 149. (You want your muscles to be warm for the Yoga and Pilates routine, so cool down after your walking workout, but don't sit down.) Finish with the Post-Workout Stretching Routine on page 129.

The Great Outdoors Workout #1

Hiking has long been an outdoor activity that many fitness enthusiasts flock to for the workout, the view, and the absence of sirens, landlords, and traffic. Adding some hiking workouts to your exercise routine is a great way to challenge yourself and burn up a huge number of calories.

The following program is one of two for hiking in nature. This one will be to prepare your body for the difficult workout that hiking often is.

For most hiking expeditions, whether it's a day trip or a week-long event, you're going to need a hiking pack. Be sure to purchase a pack that's designed to distribute the weight equally across your entire upper body, while allowing you to stand tall with relative ease. To prepare for your workout, first load up your pack so that it weighs between 10 and 15 pounds. You'll be needing your loaded-up hiking pack in just a moment.

- First, to prepare your heart, lungs, and muscles for exercise, ease in with a light warm-up of walking for 10 minutes at an easy pace. When you're finished, you'll need to return to your car or home for your hiking pack, so don't stray too far.

- Once you've completed your warm-up, strap on that loaded hiking pack. For this portion of your workout, I want you to head somewhere where there's a hill, so that you can increase the challenge of your workout. (If you live in an area that doesn't have hills, you can simulate this portion of the routine on a treadmill. More on that below.) When you get to the hill, begin walking up and down it with your weighted pack. Walk 50 to 100 yards up and then down the hill, repeating this for 15 minutes.

    Note: Because the following exercises are performed while wearing a weighted hiking pack, they're particularly challenging. Be sure the weight in your pack is distributed evenly across your back, and that you do the exercises with proper form. Do not perform these exercises if you have prior back or neck injuries. If you start to experience pain or fatigue, take all or part of the weight out of your hiking pack.

    To simulate this portion of the workout on a treadmill: Set the grade, or incline, at 1 and increase it slowly over the 15 minutes to a grade of 5. Don't walk for more than 2 minutes at a grade of 5, though, since the extra weight of your hiking pack can aggravate your lower back.

- For the next portion of our routine, find a staircase. (If you live in a town where the local high school football stadium is open to the public, this can be a perfect place for a stair workout.) Begin walking up the staircase, with your pack, taking two steps at a time, and then one step at a time on the way back down. Complete 20 sets up and down the stairs.

- Next, face sideways, so your right side is facing up the stairs, and left facing down. Place your right foot on the second step and step up to that step and return. Complete 15 reps. Then turn and repeat this move on the opposite side, leading with your left foot, for 15 reps.

- Lastly, walk on flat ground for 20 minutes, alternating every 3 minutes of walking with 30 seconds of walking lunges.

    Walking Lunge: Take a large step forward, while maintaining a tall, upright upper body. Strike the lead foot, keeping the weight on the heel and midfoot. Next, drop down by bending your back knee. Don't let your back knee touch the ground. Hold for 3 seconds. Continue with the opposite foot stepping forward.

- Bring your breathing and heart rate back down with a 5-minute cooldown, walking at one-half to one-quarter of your previous pace.
- Finish by stretching out and lengthening your muscles with the Post-Workout Stretching Routine on page 129.

    Intermediate Level: Complete the workout as described above, but do the final walking portion for 35 minutes instead of 20. Perform the 30-second walking lunge intervals every 2 minutes, instead of every 3. Be sure to finish with a 5-minute cooldown, followed by the Post-Workout Stretching Routine on page 129.

    Advanced Level: Complete the Intermediate-Level workout as described above, but add more items to your hiking pack so that it weighs up to 15 pounds. Then add in the Yoga and Pilates Routine on page 149 before completing the Post-Workout Stretching Routine.

The Great Outdoors Workout #2

The second routine for our hiking trip involves more advance movements and requires about an hour of your time. In addition to leg work, we will be focusing on balance, upper-body strength, and building endurance.

- First, to prepare your heart, lungs, and muscles for exercise, ease in with a light warm-up of walking for 10 minutes at an easy pace.
- We'll begin this routine with some strength work performed while wearing your hiking pack weighted with 10 to 15 pounds. (See note on previous page.)

    Squat Press: Find a medicine ball or an equivalent object weighing roughly 10 pounds. If you have a tent, most likely it comes in a bag. Use this! Holding the object at your upper chest with both hands, stand with your feet shoulder-width apart. Now move your hips backward and downward until your knees reach 90 degrees, then stand back up while pressing the object upward over the height of your head, but never outside your peripheral vision. Complete 20 repetitions.

Side-to-Side Lunge with a Reach and Grab Motion: This move will simulate gathering wood for building a fire. Many people injure themselves with this type of activity. It's important to maintain a strong upper-body posture to minimize the risk for a lower-back injury.

Step out to one side, sitting your hips back and downward. Next, reach out with your arms to pick up a 5-pound object (if you have a medicine ball, this is ideal), stand up with the weight, and then put the weight down on the other side. This is one rep. Repeat to the other side. Complete 10 repetitions to each side.

Push-Up: To develop a strong upper body, nothing beats this old standard. And though just about everyone *thinks* they know how to do a push-up, it's often done with improper form. Remove your pack and lie face down. Raise your body off the floor with your arms. Your palms should be flat on the floor, spaced shoulder-width apart. Your feet are positioned on their toes, and your body is straight, like a plank. Keep your eyes looking straight down at the floor and "suck in" your stomach to minimize arching of your lower back and the risk of injury to that region. Now bend your elbows and lower your body until your torso is 6 inches from the floor, or you reach a 90-degree angle at your elbow joints. Then begin to straighten your arms and raise your body upward. (To confirm that you're using proper form, check out the photo on page 140.) To keep from rushing through each push-up, count to 2 on the descent and then to 2 on the ascent. Complete 12 to 20 reps, making sure you're using good form.

If you have difficulty completing this move, begin with your knees on the ground, and follow the same movement pattern for the upper body as described above. See the photo on page 141.

• After you've completed the strength-training moves, you're now ready for the fitness walking portion of the workout. I want you to walk for 30 minutes while wearing your weighted hiking pack, as directed below.

Minutes 1 through 10: Walk at a pace of approximately 3.9 mph. Stay on relatively flat terrain.

Minutes 11 through 20: Continue at the same pace (approximately 3.9 mph), but try to tackle some hills. Because you're wearing a weighted pack, don't head straight down the hill; instead, go from one side of the hill to the other in a zigzag pattern until you reach the bottom.

Minutes 21 through 30: Increase your speed to about 4.2 to 4.3 mph. To burn even more calories, try to find a hill with a slight incline to walk up.

- Finally, bring your breathing and heart rate back down with a 5-minute cooldown, walking at one-half to one-quarter of your previous pace.
- Finish your workout by completing the Post-Workout Stretching Routine on page 129.

Intermediate Level: Increase the weight of the medicine ball or other object you use for the squat press and side-to-side lunge; for example, if you had been using a 10-pound object, use a 20-pound object instead. Do 4 sets of push-ups with 30 seconds between each set. Complete till muscles are completely fatigued. End with the 5-minute cooldown walk and the Post-Workout Stretching Routine on page 129.

Advanced Level: Complete the Intermediate-Level workout as described above, but add more items to your hiking pack so that it weighs up to 25 pounds. Then complete the Yoga and Pilates Routine on page 149 before doing the Post-Workout Stretching Routine.

Now and Later: Erase Pounds with Short Bursts of Exercise

The great thing about weight loss and the human body is that the human body doesn't keep records of when you worked out or how much you did. All the body wants to know is "How much energy will you need for this activity, and where do you want it to come from?" If you're pressed for time (and who isn't these days?), consider the following routine, which allows you to break up your workout time into short workouts throughout the day.

What's more, science not only supports, but encourages, breaking up your workouts. For example, in a study at Loughborough University in Leicestershire, England, researchers found that women who walked continuously for 30 minutes 5 days a week had almost identical increases in fitness as women who split their 30 minutes into three 10-minute walks. Perhaps even more encouraging was that the women who took short walks lost more weight and reported greater decreases in waist circumference than the women who took long walks.

Here are a few ways to get your 30 minutes of walking in today. Before each mini-workout, warm up your muscles by walking at an easy pace for a few minutes.

- **Crack of Dawn:** If you are a parent or have an early morning regimen, then it's probably very difficult to get to the gym before the kids wake or the work whistle sings. A 10-minute walk either on the treadmill or around the block is a great way to start any day. It will not only burn calories, but it will jump-start your metabolism and give you energy for the rest of the day.

With a treadmill: Set the incline at 6 degrees and walk at 4 mph for 10 minutes.

Outdoors: As you walk around the block, search for a hill or a set of stairs to add the natural resistance of gravity. Walk swiftly for 10 minutes.

- **Lunch Break:** When we're knee deep in work due yesterday, lunch breaks are often diminished to a packed lunch at our desks. Some people will actually use their lunch break to work out, but then have very little time to eat!

  If you work in a building where there is a fitness facility, take full advantage of this opportunity to get your appetite ready for lunch and an energy boost to finish off your workday ahead.

  With a treadmill: Set the incline at 6 degrees and walk at 4 mph for 10 minutes.

  Without a treadmill: Take the stairs to start your workout. If the weather is not being supportive, this is where your workout will stay for the next 10 minutes. Walking up and down stairs for 10 minutes will burn super amounts of calories. Likewise, if you can get outside, try to find some hills to walk up and down, which will increase the number of calories you burn.

- **Dinnertime:** Let's skip that dessert and treat your body to the healthiest conclusion to any day: exercise.

  To complete your day, take a 10-minute after-dinner walk around your neighborhood or walk in place in your living room for the same amount of time. Even though they may last only a few minutes, frequent bursts of exercise over the course of a day improve circulation, build heart and lung strength, and burn extra calories. Alternatively, complete 10 minutes on your treadmill, with the same intensity as above. Congratulations, you do have the time to get fit!

- Finish your day by completing the Post-Workout Stretching Routine on page 129. Not only will it lengthen and stretch out the muscles you've just used, but it will relax you and help you mentally put away the stresses of the day for a relaxing evening.

  Intermediate Level: Complete the exercise sessions as described above, but double your walking time to 20 minutes each time and increase your pace to a brisk walk of 4.5 mph. You'll more than double the number of calories you burn! End with the Post-Workout Stretching Routine on page 129.

Advanced Level: Complete the exercise sessions as described in the Intermediate-Level workout. Don't forget to end with the Post-Workout Stretching Routine on page 129. In addition, complete the Yoga and Pilates Routine on page 149 and the Post-Workout Stretching Routing (on page 129) at whatever time you can work it in during the course of your day.

Heart Healthy

I'm not a fan of scare tactics, but heart disease is still the nation's leading cause of death. According to the American College of Sports Medicine and the American Dietetic Association, there are several established risk factors for heart disease. They are cigarette smoking, hypertension, high cholesterol, impaired fasting glucose, obesity, a sedentary lifestyle, and family history.

The good news is that 6 out of these 7 risk factors are within your control. If you smoke, you need to talk with your doctor *today* about quitting. Regular physical activity and a healthy diet can take care of and correct the next five factors—hypertension (also known as high blood pressure), high cholesterol, impaired fasting glucose, obesity, and a sedentary lifestyle.

Family history is the one exception to the rule, but even here, there is good news. In addition to noting any immediate blood relatives (parents, siblings, and children) who passed away prematurely (considered to be under 55 years old for males or under 65 years old for females), look at how these people lived. Did they themselves have the above risk factors, and if so, why did they? Was there something about their lifestyle that increased their risk for these factors and, ultimately, for heart disease? If so, and if you have corrected these unhealthy factors in your own lifestyle, you have likely significantly decreased your heart disease risk.

Finally, get a physical, preferably one that includes a Bruce protocol stress test. And be sure to talk to your physician about your lifestyle and any risk factors you have so that you can gain a better understanding of their role in your life.

Current recommendations for cardiovascular health (pertaining to your heart, lungs, and blood systems) are to complete moderate physical activity most days of the week. Moderate physical activity is any form of exercise that you can maintain for 30 minutes a day, and breaking that up into two or three separate workouts is just fine, too. In fact, consistent, moderate physical activity is the only proven method to decrease bad cholesterol (LDL) and increase good cholesterol (HDL). Whether you're on a treadmill, at the park, or strolling through your neighborhood, moderate physical activity on most days of the week will decrease your risk for cardiovascular disease.

The following workout routine allows you to use your target heart rate zone as a training tool. By monitoring it, you'll be able to measure how hard your body is working. For this workout routine, we're going to designate 50 to 75 percent of your maximum heart rate as your target heart rate zone. (You'll recall from "Get in the Zone" on page 49 that you should never work out at your maximum heart rate, which is calculated by subtracting your age from 220. Instead, the target heart rate zone is calculated by figuring out percentages of it.)

- First, to prepare your heart, lungs, and muscles for exercise, ease in with a light warm-up of walking for 10 minutes at an easy pace.
- Next, I want you to complete 30 minutes of walking, either outside or on a treadmill. During these 30 minutes, try to stay within your target heart rate zone. When you first begin my exercise program, try to stay at the low end of your target heart rate zone, at about the 50 to 55 percent range. After you've been working on my programs for about 6 weeks, you can walk for the 30 minutes at gradually higher levels within your target heart rate zone.

  To stay within your target heart rate zone, you'll need to take your pulse during your fitness walks. For the most accurate read, find your pulse at the side of your neck (at the carotid artery). Put your first 2 fingers over your pulse and count the number of beats within a 10-second period. Then multiply this number by 6, and you'll have your number of heartbeats in a minute. For example, if you counted your pulse to be 20 during the 10-second pulse count, your heart rate would be 120 beats per minute. For an easier read on your pulse, purchase a heart rate monitor, preferably one with a chest strap. (See "Resources" on page 172 for recommendations.)

- Now bring your breathing and heart rate back down with a 5-minute cooldown, walking at one-half to one-quarter of your previous pace.
- Finish your workout by completing the Post-Workout Stretching Routine on page 129.

Target Heart Rates by Age

HEARTBEATS PER MINUTE (percent of maximum heart rate)

Age	Low (50%)	High (75%)
20	100	150
25	98	146
30	95	143
35	93	139
40	90	135
45	88	131
50	85	128
55	83	124
60	80	120
65	78	116
70	75	113
75	73	109
80	70	105

Note: If you are taking certain medications, such as beta blockers, you may not be able to reach your target heart rate. Always have your doctor's permission before beginning any exercise program.

Intermediate Level: Increase your walking time to 45 minutes at gradually increasing levels of your target heart rate zone. End with the 5-minute cooldown walk and the Post-Workout Stretching Routine on page 129.

Advanced Level: Complete the Intermediate-Level workout as described above, walking for 45 minutes at or near the upper limit of your target heart rate zone (75 percent of your maximum heart rate). Then complete the Yoga and Pilates Routine on page 149 before doing the Post-Workout Stretching Routine.

No Joint Pain Necessary

More than 40 million people in the United States—or one out of every six—has some form of arthritis. The term *arthritis* is used to describe a disorder of one or more joints. Arthritis disorders are actually part of a broader group of disorders of the muscles and bones called *musculoskeletal disorders*. Three of the most commonly occurring musculoskeletal conditions are osteoarthritis, rheumatoid arthritis, and osteoporosis. Osteoarthritis is one of the most common forms of arthritis and is caused by the gradual wear and tear of joints over time. On the other hand, rheumatoid arthritis, or RA, is an autoimmune disorder and is the most crippling form of arthritis. RA affects approximately 2.1 million people in the United States, and two to three times more women than men.

Needless to say, arthritis can be a debilitating condition. The pain it may cause is often described as excruciating and can dramatically affect the style of living you have grown to love in your youngest years.

Fortunately, there is good news. A regular exercise program may help relieve the pain—and even help to prevent the disease in the first place. In order to understand why arthritis can be so painful—and why exercise can help—you need to understand the basic anatomy of a joint. While many people think joints are simply places where two bones meet, they are more complex than this. In addition to the two bones that meet at a joint, each joint is supported by muscles, tendons, and ligaments. Each joint also includes padding, namely cartilage, which cushions the joint and decreases the impact of natural forces, allowing the articulation of the joint to be smooth, rhythmic, and pain-free. In many cases, joint pain is solely an inflammation of these misunderstood structures. But why does this happen? Joint mobility and ability are mostly determined by the condition and function of the muscles that surround the joint. Let's take the knee, for example. An amazing construction of ligaments, bony articulations, tendons, muscles, and lots of padding allows you to take several thousand steps a day for an average of 80 years. That's a lot of work for your knees.

In my experience, some knee and other joint problems originate from muscular changes that are a result of simply being active over the years. We all seem to have a slight imbalance somewhere in our bodies: too strong on one side, too weak on the other, lack of or excessive flexibility in one muscle group, and lack thereof in the opposing group. Maybe a sport we play has overworked one muscle group, putting stress on another group of muscles. All joints are about a harmony and balance of the musculature. Any deviation from a perfectly balanced body will impose forces on our ligaments and muscles. So, how can we create this harmony? For strong joints, we need a balance of strength and flexibility in the muscles surrounding them.

This exercise routine combines calorie-burning walking (an activity that's naturally easy on the joints) with special body-weight exercises to help prevent joint pain.

- First, to prepare your heart, lungs, and muscles for exercise, ease in with a light warm-up of walking for 10 minutes at an easy pace.
- Next, if no pain is present, pick up your pace to a brisk walk at 3.5 mph and complete 30 minutes of walking at this pace.
- Complete the walking portion of the workout with a 5-minute cooldown walk at one-half to one-quarter of your previous pace.
- Now it's time for the strength-training portion of the workout. Remember: By strengthening the muscles around your joints, you can also improve joint strength and limit any pain.

Squat Press: Using both hands, hold a medicine ball or other object weighing roughly 10 pounds at upper-chest level. Stand with your feet shoulder-width apart. Keeping the ball at your chest, move your hips backward and downward, as if you were sitting in a chair, until your knees reach 90 degrees. Then stand back up while pressing the ball upward over the height of your head, but never outside your peripheral vision. Don't let the ball travel behind your head. Complete 2 sets of 25 reps each.

Walking Lunge: Take a large step forward, while maintaining a tall, upright upper body. Strike the lead foot, keeping the weight on the heel and mid-foot. Next, drop down by bending your back knee. Don't let your back knee touch the floor. Pause at the bottom, and then stand back up by lifting your back leg as you travel down the hallway or sidewalk. Your hands and arms can be by your side, or wherever you feel balanced, but don't place them on your legs for assistance. Continue for 30 seconds.

Push-Up: Lie face down, with your hands and feet below you, supporting your body in a fixed position, creating a plank with your body. Your palms should be flat on the floor, spaced shoulder-width apart. Your feet are positioned on their toes, and your body is straight. "Suck in" your stomach to minimize arching of your lower back. Next, bend your elbows and lower your body to a point roughly 6 inches from the ground. Then raise your body back up. To keep from rushing through each push-up, count to 2 on the descent and then to 2 on the ascent. Complete as many reps as possible, until muscle failure. If you have difficulty completing this move, begin with your knees on the ground, and follow the same movement pattern for the upper body as described above. To make sure you're using proper form, see the photos on page 140.

Jumping Jack: Start with your arms down at your sides and your feet together, with your back straight. As you jump a few inches off the floor, extend your arms over your head in a wide circular path. As you raise your arms, spread your legs until your feet are slightly wider than shoulder-width apart. Bring your arms down as you jump to bring your legs back together. Complete five 1-minute intervals.

Hamstring Curl with Physioball: Lie on your back on the floor, with your legs slightly flexed and positioned atop a physioball. Press your heels into the north pole of the ball. Next, press into the ball with your legs, raising your torso off the floor. Lift your hips until they cannot raise themselves any further. Your arms should be by your sides at all times, and your head and shoulders should be relaxed and against the floor. As you reach the top position of the lift, begin to curl your legs beneath your thighs, bringing your heels inward. Be sure to maintain the full hip lift while curling in. Do 3 sets of 15 reps each. To make sure you're using proper form, see the photo on page 144.

Seated Row with Exercise Tubing: Wrap the exercise tubing around a sturdy pole, door, or doorknob. Sit about 4 feet away on the floor, with your feet extended and knees slightly bent. Grab the exercise tubing with both hands. Keeping your lower back erect, pull the tubing until it's tight, bringing your hands and arms from an extended position back into your body-your elbows should be close to your rib cage and the tubing should land at your lower chest. Complete 3 sets of 25 reps each.

• Finish your workout by completing the Post-Workout Stretching Routine on page 129. This will stretch out and lengthen the muscles you've just worked.

Intermediate Level: Do the workout as described above, but complete the last two exercises twice (so that you're doing six sets of each), with a set of jumping jacks for 2 minutes between each set. Finish with the Post-Workout Stretching Routine on page 129.

Advanced Level: Complete the Intermediate-Level workout as described above, but add in the Yoga and Pilates Routine on page 149 before completing the Post-Workout Stretching Routine.

Business and Vacation Travel

In today's global economy, business and travel are often considered contingent upon each other. Each day, millions of Americans board planes, hop on trains, or hit the highways in their cars on business trips. In order to remain healthy and active, we must find a way to support our regular exercise routine even when business takes us away from home.

And while most of us look forward to some well-deserved R&R when we travel for pleasure, vacations can be the perfect time to jump-start or add a new dimension to a workout routine. Exercising in a new environment—away from the stresses and responsibilities of our daily lives—can rejuvenate our spirits and motivate us to continue working out when we get home.

The first step is to pack the items we'll need to maintain our workout routine. Use the following list as you pack your bags.

☐ Athletic apparel that does not include the use of natural fibers such as cotton. Choose newer fibers made of polyester, fleece, or wools, which will keep you comfortable and dry under all conditions indoors and out.

☐ Lightweight athletic shoes with a flexible upper lining construction to allow for easy packing in a suitcase.

☐ Performance socks that don't have cotton in the blend of fibers. Also, look for socks that have reinforced Lycra webbings around the midfoot. This design adds additional support and comfort in the arch and midfoot.

☐ Plenty of water. Be sure to take along some bottled water, especially if you're traveling on an airplane. Dehydration is accelerated during air travel and can make workouts later that day more difficult and less effective. The human body can absorb 8 ounces of water per hour on average and will lose much more than that during exercise. So, do the numbers and get hydrated!

☐ Exercise tubing. It can provide hundreds of pounds of resistance if so desired, but it weighs only a few ounces. Check out your local fitness equipment retailer to purchase this handy travel workout tool!

If you're in a hotel building, refer to the Now and Later workout on page 103 for an exercise routine you can do indoors without a gym.

If you're vacationing by an ocean or lake, read the Hit the Beach workout presented on page 119 for a heart-pumping routine.

Enjoy your healthier travel time.

Getting a Workout When You're Far from Home

I work in the fitness industry and must travel frequently. In addition to business travels, my family is scattered throughout the United States and Europe, and I have relatives as far away as Papua, New Guinea. (One time, I hiked the highlands of this remote Pacific island to get my workout.) I've interviewed a lot of business (and leisure) travelers along the way, and I know I'm not alone when I say that getting a decent workout when you're traveling can be difficult.

Fortunately, I've picked up some useful information through my travels that has made working out while away from home much easier. Here are some tips to help health-conscious, busy travelers get their exercise while on the road:

Read all about it. I recommend picking up a copy of *Hotel Gyms: The Fitness Guide,* by Kyle Merker (Incline Press, 1997). This paperback book rates fitness facilities in 45 U.S. cities and at all the major hotel chains, describing the specific equipment at each location, such as how many treadmills there really are in that hotel gym.

Go online. City Sport Worldwide (www. cityguide.com) is a guide to sports and leisure activities in cities around the globe. In Seattle, for example, hiking day trips range from easy to moderate treks just north of the city to more challenging destinations. Or check out www.airportgyms .com for airport gyms or facilities near your hotels destinations.

Find a gym. For information about fitness facilities at YMCAs or YWCAs, visit their web sites www.ywca.org and www.ymca.net. Also, if you belong to a local gym that has sites in other cities, find out if it has "passport" memberships or offers discounts to gyms in the city you are traveling to.

Take advantage of your hotel's facilities. One hotel chain that usually offers superior fitness facilities is the Four Seasons group. The luxury hotel chain even has a toll-free phone number and a Web site that allows you to get specific information about a particular hotel's fitness center and whether it offers certified personal trainers. Even if you're not staying with this hotel chain, though, be sure to ask about your hotel's fitness facilities when booking your room. Also inquire about any local parks that have walking trails.

The following workout includes strength-training exercises and stretches that are easily portable for wherever your port of call. I send my clients out the door with instructions to pack their exercise tubes, jump rope, walking shoes, and the discipline to fit in these exercises. I want you to do the same.

Before you book your hotel, check with the concierge for information on local parks that include walking trails. Or pick up a map of the city you'll be visiting and plan a walk that will allow you to do a bit of sightseeing along the way. (If you're on vacation, rather than a business trip, and plan to do a lot of sightseeing, I recommend wearing a pedometer so that you can count your steps.)

- First, to prepare your heart, lungs, and muscles for exercise, ease in with a light warm-up of walking for 10 minutes at an easy pace.
- Next, complete a 30-minute fitness walk at a pace of 3.5 to 4 mph.
- Complete the walking portion of the workout with a 5-minute cooldown walk at one-half to one-quarter of your previous pace as you return to your hotel room.
- Now it's time for the strength-training portion of the workout. All of the following exercises can easily be done in your hotel room, state room, or even a cabin car.

> **Jumping Jack:** Warm up by doing 20 to 30 jumping jacks. If you haven't done this old standard in a while, here's a refresher: Start with your arms down at your sides and your feet together, with your back straight. As you jump a few inches off the floor, extend your arms over your head in a wide circular path. As you raise your arms, spread your legs until your feet are slightly wider than shoulder-width apart. Bring your arms down as you jump to bring your legs back together.

> **Push-Up:** After completing the jumping jacks, move right in to your push-ups: Raise your body off the floor with your arms. Your palms should be flat on the floor, spaced shoulder-width apart. Your feet are positioned on their toes, and your body is straight, like a plank. Keep your eyes looking straight down at the floor, and "suck in" your stomach to minimize arching of your lower back and the risk of injury to that region. Now bend your elbows and lower your body until your torso is 6 inches from the floor, or you reach a 90-degree angle at your elbow joints. Then begin to straighten your arms and raise your body upward. (To confirm that you're using proper form, check out the photo on page 140.) To keep from rushing through each push-up,

count to 2 on the descent and then to 2 on the ascent. Complete 3 sets of 15 to 20 reps each.

Note: If you have difficulty completing this move, begin with your knees on the ground, and follow the same movement pattern for the upper body as described above. See the photo on page 140.

Stationary Squat with Tubing: Stand with the tubing around your ankles, or place both feet lightly on it. Move your feet slightly wider than shoulder-width apart, bearing the majority of the weight on your heels. Next sit your hips backward away from your body, while keeping your eyes and chin up at a 45-degree angle relative to the ground. With your arms out in front of you, holding the ends of the tubing, begin to perform a sitting move until your knees have reached an angle of about 90 degrees, but never more than that. Keep your back in a neutral position, never arched. One repetition should take about 5 seconds (2 seconds descending, 1 second pause, and 2 seconds ascending). Complete 3 sets of 15 to 20 reps each.

Side-to-Side Lunge: Place your feet a wide distance apart. Point your toes forward. Place your hands above your knees. Bend your right knee, keeping your left leg straight. Your torso should be in as upright a position as possible—try not to lean forward. Go down as low as you can without strain, being sure to keep your knees in line with your toes. If you'd like, you can hold on to a chair for support as you go down and up to help keep your torso upright. Come up and repeat on the other side. Complete 3 sets of 15 to 20 reps each.

Wall Squat: Stand about 12 to 18 inches away from a wall, with your back to the wall. Squat down, bending at the knees and lowering your hips no lower than knee level. Keep your knees behind your toes, and your back leaning against the wall. Hold the squat for 10 seconds, then stand up pressing through your heels. Complete 3 sets of 15 to 20 reps each.

Static Front Lunge: Stand with your feet shoulder-width apart. Step forward with one leg, keeping your front knee in line with your toes. Lift your chest (without arching your back), and bend your back knee, but don't allow it to touch the floor. Keep your front knee at or above a 90-degree angle. Exhale, lift your body, and return to your starting position. Repeat with the opposite leg. Complete 3 sets of 15 to 20 reps each.

Seated Row with Exercise Tubing: Wrap the exercise tubing around a doorknob. Sit about 4 feet away on the floor, with your feet extended and knees slightly bent. Grab the exercise tubing with both hands. Keeping your lower back erect, pull the tubing until it's tight, bringing your hands and arms from an extended position back into your body. Your elbows should be close to your rib cage and the tubing should land at your lower chest. Complete 3 sets of 15 to 20 reps each.

- Finish your workout by completing the Post-Workout Stretching Routine on page 129. This routine is also easily done in a small space, and it will stretch out and lengthen the muscles you've just worked.

Intermediate Level: Do the workout as described above, but increase the fitness walk to 45 minutes at 4 to 4.5 mph. Finish with the Post-Workout Stretching Routine on page 129.

Advanced Level: Complete the workout as described above, but increase the fitness walk to a full hour at 4 to 5 mph. Add in the Yoga and Pilates Routine on page 149 before completing the Post-Workout Stretching Routine.

The Post-Pregnancy or Post-Surgery Workout

If you're a new (or even not so new) mom, you may be having a hard time losing the weight you gained during your pregnancy. And if you had a C-section, you may be a little nervous about starting an exercise routine. Similarly, if you've had surgery in the past few weeks, you may be getting antsy to get out of the house and get moving once again.

The good news is that gentle exercise will likely make you feel better, help in your recovery, and—if you're battling pregnancy weight—burn extra calories. The following workout is designed to take into account your special needs. Before beginning it, however, be sure to get your doctor's okay. Most physicians recommend 8 to 12 weeks of recovery time for most surgery before beginning an exercise program.

The first order of business when beginning an exercise program after, say, knee surgery or having a baby by Caesarean section is to establish fundamental, functional movements. No additional resistance outside of your own body weight is required at this time.

- First, to prepare your heart, lungs, and muscles for exercise, ease in with a light warm-up of walking for 10 minutes at an easy pace.

• Next, complete the following three exercises in a circuit five times. Your rest periods should not exceed 1 minute.

Step-Up: Find a sturdy staircase or a makeshift step about 8 inches tall that will support your body weight. Step up onto the stair or box leading with your right foot and follow the right with the left until both feet have ascended together. (As you step up, lead with your heel and be sure to keep your knees in line with your toes on top of the step.) Step down with the right and then the left foot. Repeat this exercise for 1 minute, leading for the first 30 seconds with your right foot and the second 30 seconds with your left.

¾-Depth Squat: Standing with your feet shoulder-width apart, complete a ¾-depth squat. Maintain upper-body posture that is similar to standing erect. Keep your arms straight out in front of your body. This exercise is crucial because your abdominals will begin to contract to balance and stabilize your spine. This is the first step in rebuilding the strength and stability of your abdominal musculature, something that is particularly important if you've given birth recently. Repeat this exercise for 1 minute.

Walking Lunge: A walking lunge is an excellent way to stretch and strengthen the muscles of the legs and abdominal complex. Again, upper-body posture dictates the efficacy of the total movement. Take a large step forward, while maintaining a tall, upright upper body. Strike the lead foot, keeping the weight on the heel and midfoot. Next, drop down by bending your back knee, but don't let it touch the floor. Pause at the bottom, then stand back up by lifting your back leg as you travel down your hallway or sidewalk. Your hands and arms can be by your sides, or wherever you feel balanced, but don't place them onto your legs for assistance. Complete for 1 minute.

• After completing the circuit five times, it's now time to start walking. Walk at a slow, comfortable, 3 mph pace for 15 minutes, avoiding hills. If you have access to a treadmill, I recommend doing your walk on it, since the soft surface will be gentle on your body.

• Bring your breathing and heart rate back down with a 5-minute cooldown, walking at a gentle, slow pace.

• Finish your workout by completing the Post-Workout Stretching Routine on page 129.

Note: Because this is a recovery workout, there are no intermediate- or advanced-level versions of it. When this workout becomes easy for you, you'll know that your physical fitness and endurance have improved. Discuss your progress with your doctor. When he or she believes you are ready, you can then move on to the more challenging programs in this book.

Baby, Stroller, and You

So, you've got the kids, the spouse, and one or more full-time jobs. Chances are, time is a rare commodity in your home. And when you do have time for a workout, you may not want to leave your kids with your spouse or other caregiver. That's why I've designed the following workout, which allows you to push your baby in a stroller at the same time you get a fabulous workout. Plus, the additional workload of pushing that stroller will increase the intensity of the workout, thus burning more calories!

If you're in a park, you can easily do this workout on grassy off-road surfaces. The additional resistance will increase the workload even further.

There are a few important things to keep in mind before you complete the following stroller workout.

- Posture is often compromised during this activity. Be sure to stand up straight as you walk, with your shoulders down and back, not hunched over. Try to contract your abs as you push the stroller.
- Don't lean on the stroller, which could add undue stress to the shoulder complex and spinal column.
- Remember to keep your eyes forward at all times.
- Take breaks every 5 minutes to check in on the passenger of your stroller, catch your breath, check your posture, and map out the next segment of your workout!
- Be sure to pack plenty of water, snacks, changes of diapers, and the appropriate clothing.
- Remember sunscreen for yourself and your children.
- Dress appropriately with performance athletic apparel. And remember that even though you may get warm as you do the workout, your child isn't getting the exercise you are, so be sure he or she is dressed appropriately.

  Ready to begin? The following fitness walk will take you approximately 30 minutes, all of which is spent with your baby safely nestled in the stroller.

- First, to prepare your heart, lungs, and muscles for exercise, ease in with a light warm-up of walking and pushing the stroller for 5 minutes at an easy pace. Stay on mostly flat terrain.
- Next, find a hill that takes about 1 minute to walk up. Walk up and down this hill pushing your stroller and baby 5 times. For safety's sake, don't head straight down the hill; instead, go from one side of the hill to the other in a zigzag pattern until you reach the bottom. This portion of the workout should take about 10 minutes total.
- Next, find some more flat terrain and walk for 5 minutes.
- When the 5 minutes are up, stop and do 3 sets of 15 squats. Keep one hand on the stroller for balance. (*Note:* Be sure to lock the wheels on the stroller before beginning your squats!) Rest for 30 seconds between each set. This should take approximately 5 minutes.

  Squat: Stand with your feet slightly wider than shoulder-width apart, bearing the majority of the weight on your heels and not on the stroller. Place one hand lightly on the stroller for balance and sit your hips backward away from your body, while keeping your eyes and chin up at a 45-degree angle relative to the ground. Begin to perform a sitting move until your knees have reached an angle of about 90 degrees, but never more than that. Keep your back in a neutral position, never arched. One repetition should take about 5 seconds (2 seconds descending, 1 second pause, and 2 seconds ascending).

  Note: If your baby wakes up when you stop pushing the stroller, get him or her out of the stroller to help you with your squats. The additional weight helps you burn calories; plus, this will be bonding fun for you and your baby! (It's never too soon to set a good example when it comes to fitness.)

- Finally, complete 5 more minutes of walking on flat terrain at one-half to one-quarter of your previous pace. This slow-paced cooldown walk will safely bring down your breathing and heart rate.
- When you're back at home, complete the Post-Workout Stretching Routine on page 129. This will stretch out and lengthen the muscles you've just worked.

  Intermediate Level: Double your time spent on each portion of the fitness walk and double your calories. It's that easy! Don't forget to complete the Post-Workout Stretching Routine on page 129 when you return home.

Advanced Level: Complete the Intermediate-Level workout as described above, but add in the Yoga and Pilates Routine on page 149 before completing the Post-Workout Stretching Routine.

Hit the Beach!

The beach is a great place to relax, but it's also a terrific place to enjoy an outdoor workout, barefoot! Plus, the sand provides resistance for strengthening the muscles of the feet and ankles in ways you can't when you're walking on pavement or solid ground. The uneven surface challenges your feet to adapt with every step of fresh terrain. If you're lucky enough to live next to a beach, take frequent advantage of the exercise opportunities it provides. And if you find that you're starting to get bored with your exercise routine and you live within a reasonable driving distance from an ocean or lake, doing a beach workout in the early mornings, evenings, or on the weekend can inspire and rejuvenate you. But even if your home is far from an ocean or lake, you can still use this workout on your next vacation to the shore.

Note: If you have weak ankles, complete this exercise routine with your shoes on.

- To prepare your heart, lungs, and muscles for exercise, ease in with a light warm-up of walking for 10 minutes at an easy pace (either on a sidewalk or in hard sand). Begin your workout by walking close to the water, but not in the water or surf. The sand in this area is generally packed down firmly and will allow you to walk for extended periods of time. Remain on the firm sand close to the surf for the first 10 minutes. Remember to keep your eyes and chin up to avoid slouching your upper body. It's easy to break posture when the terrain is uneven and as soft as sand can be.

- For the next 10 minutes, alternate between walking for 50 yards at a time in the firm sand and then 50 yards in the softer sand further from the shore. Repeat these 50-yard intervals until the 10 minutes are completed.

- For the last 10 minutes, I want you to walk into and out of the immediate surf (in water 8 to 20 inches deep). Once again, make these intervals 50 yards long at a time, switching from the shoreline sand to the immediate surf. The added resistance of the surf will increase the intensity of the exercise. Avoid walking deeper than knee depth. Lifting your legs out of the deeper water too often can cause other muscles of the hip region to tighten from overuse.

- Following your fitness walk, cool down by walking in the hard sand for 5 minutes at one-half to one-quarter of your previous pace.

- To stretch out your calves after this challenging workout, do this calf stretch.

  Calf Stretch: Find a stair or curb to stand on and extend your heels off the back. If needed, you can balance your upper body by holding onto a railing or wall. Stretch each leg by alternately lowering the heel below the level of the stair. Keep your knee on the extended leg soft, not locked. Hold each stretch for 20 to 30 seconds. Do 5 reps on each leg, being careful not to bounce.

- Once you've stretched out your calf muscles, turn your attention to stretching out the rest of your body with the Post-Workout Stretching Routine on page 129.

  Intermediate Level: After completing a warm-up walk of 10 minutes at an easy pace (either on a sidewalk or in hard sand), complete the following workout.

  Minutes 1 to 10: Walk on the firm sand close to the surf.

  Minutes 11 to 30: Alternate between walking for 100 yards at a time in the firm sand and then 100 yards in the softer sand further from the shore. Repeat these 100-yard intervals until the 20 minutes are completed.

  Minutes 31 to 50: Complete 100-yard intervals walking on the firm shoreline sand alternating with walking in the immediate surf (in water 8 to 20 inches deep). Do not walk in water higher than your knees. Repeat until the 20 minutes are completed.

  Finish with a 5-minute cooldown by walking in hard sand at one-half to one-quarter of your previous pace.

  Complete 5 reps with each leg of the calf stretch, as described above. Follow this with the Post-Workout Stretching Routine on page 129.

  Advanced Level: Complete the Intermediate-Level workout explained above, but add in the Yoga and Pilates Routine on page 149 before completing the Post-Workout Stretching Routine.

Winter Wonderland

Even though it's below freezing outside and school has been cancelled because of snow, there's still a workout for you in the winter wonderland that is your local park.

Before you lace up your shoes, though, give some careful consideration to your workout apparel. Insulated base layers made of fleece, coupled with stretchy mid and outer layers for comfortable fit and movement, will keep you warm and dry. Remember, cotton is for bedroom linens only. For your feet, consider socks made of merino wool, which provide adequate warmth and keep your feet dry, too.

And speaking of your feet…you can certainly do the following workout in your regular walking shoes (assuming the trails in your local park have been cleared of snow) or boots, but for a truly unique workout, try snowshoes. They'll add a totally new dimension to your workout, allowing you to wander not in the snow, but above it. Most specialty sporting goods stores offer snowshoes as well as skis, boots, and other winter gear that you can rent by the day, week, or season. Tubbs is a brand I recommend (www.tubbssnowshoes.com).

- To prepare your heart, lungs, and muscles for exercise, ease in with a light warm-up of walking indoors (either in place or on a treadmill, set at 0 grade) for 10 minutes at an easy pace.
- Next, complete the following exercises, which will work away those mid-winter blahs and gear your muscles for the challenging walk ahead.

    Wall Squat with a Ball: Stand upright next to a wall, facing away from it. Hold your physioball comfortably against the wall, in the middle of your back. Descend until your thighs are just past parallel to the floor. Extend your knees and hips until your legs are straight. Return to upright and repeat. Complete 3 sets of 12 to 15 reps each.

    Side-to-Side Lunge: Place your feet a wide distance apart. Point your toes forward. Place your hands above your knees. Bend your right knee, keeping your left leg straight. Your torso should be in as upright a position as possible; try not to lean forward. Go down as low as you can without strain, being sure to keep your knees in line with your toes. If you'd like, you can hold on to a chair for support as you go down and up to help keep your torso upright. Come up and repeat on the other side. Repeat 10 times.

    Advanced Side Lunge: While holding the end of a 3- to 5-pound dumbbell in each hand in front of your chest, palms in, raise your right knee to hip height. Contract your abdominal muscles, keeping your chest lifted and shoulders relaxed. Keeping your left leg straight, step sideways with your right foot, bending your right knee and turning your right foot out slightly so the knee and foot are aligned. Sit into your right hip, back straight, and extend the dumbbell toward the outside of your right ankle. Push off with your right foot and lift your right knee back to hip height, bringing the dumbbell to the starting position. Do 1 set of 12 lunges on each side.

• Next, put on those snowshoes (if you're using them) and head out to your local park or hiking trails for a 30- to 40-minute walk. If your park has hills, by all means, take them. This will add intensity to your workout, which means you'll burn more calories. At each 10-minute interval, stop and complete 25 squats, as described below.

Squat: Stand with your feet slightly wider than shoulder-width apart, with the weight on your heels. Next sit your hips backward away from your body, while keeping your eyes and chin up at a 45-degree angle relative to the ground. With your arms out in front of you, begin to perform a sitting move until your knees have reached an angle of about 90 degrees, but never more than that. One repetition should take about 5 seconds (2 seconds descending, 1 second pause, and 2 seconds ascending).

• Finish your walk with a 5-minute cooldown at one-half to one-quarter of your previous pace as you return to the warmth of your home.

• Once inside, I'd like you to wrap up your workout with the following move.

Static Front Lunge: Step forward with one leg, keeping your front knee in line with your toes. Lift your chest (without arching your back), and bend your back knee, but don't allow it to touch the floor. Keep your front knee at or above a 90-degree angle. Exhale, lift your body, and return to your starting position. Repeat for 10 to 12 reps with that leg. Switch the forward leg and complete another 10 to 12 reps. Perform a total of 3 sets with each leg.

• Finish your workout with the Post-Workout Stretching Routine on page 129.

Intermediate Level: Complete the workout as directed above, but do the walking portion for 1 hour and do the squats every 5 minutes instead of every 10 minutes. Finish with the cooldown, 3 sets of static front lunges, and the Post-Workout Stretching Routine on page 129.

Advanced Level: Complete the Intermediate-Level workout explained above. After completing 3 sets of static front lunges, do the Yoga and Pilates Routine found on page 149. (You want your muscles to be warm for the Yoga and Pilates routine, so cool down after your walking workout, but don't sit down.) Finish with the Post-Workout Stretching Routine on page 129.

Family Fitness

A recent study by researchers at the Johns Hopkins School of Medicine found that 93 percent of children in the United States between the ages of 8 and 17 spend several hours a day watching TV or playing video games, increasing their odds of becoming sedentary and overweight as adults. This alarming statistic should be a wake-up call for us all.

Interestingly, the National Institute of Child Health and Human Development suggests that children over the age of 2 should get 60 minutes of moderate physical activity daily for the greatest health benefit. They report that weight-bearing exercise such as walking or hiking (an activity that relies on the feet and legs carrying your weight), helps children build strong bones, strengthens their hearts, and reduces their risk for being overweight as adults.

Although I've been in the health and fitness industry for many years, I continue to marvel by what I've learned about physical activity from my sons (Lucas, age 3, and Nicholas, age 2). When it comes to getting physical, creativity comes naturally to all children. Spending active time with my sons has given me a true appreciation for the "natural fun" of movement.

My husband and I have tons of help when it comes to keeping our kids active. My parents walk, climb trees, take trips to the jungle gym, and put in CDs designed to get kids dancing and moving. Strolls in the park, time at the playground, or teaching them to garden and hike trails are a few activities my parents do to keep my sons' interest. At the beach, they'll walk for miles to watch the crabs dart in and out of the water and sand. Most of the time you can find us hanging out in the yard, digging in the dirt, riding bikes, pushing wagons, and kicking a soccer ball.

All the activities my husband and I have introduced to our children emphasize "play," rather than competition. (This is what The American Academy of Pediatrics, or AAP, recommends for children under 6 years.) We'll introduce them to organized sports later, when they reach school age. At that age, they'll be better able to handle team sports and will appreciate and enjoy the increased activity.

We even include physical fitness in many of our nightly prayers. The following poem was written for our boys by exercise physiologist and our good friend Michael Yardis.

Thank you for my jumping rope.
Thank you for my skiing slope.

Thank you for my mystery clues.
Thank you for my dancing shoes.

Thank you for my hiking trails.
Thank you for my hammer and nails.

Thank you for my wooden sleigh.
Thank you for this sunny day.

Thank you for my prancing horse.
Thank you for my putt-putt course.

Thank you for my swimming cap.
Thank you for my power nap.

Thank you for my skipping rocks.
Thank you for my fishing docks.

Thank you for my walking stick.
Thank you for my treat or trick.

Thank you for my flying kite.
Thank you for this starry night.

Thank you for my hide and seek.
Thank you for my active week.

Thank you for my bats and balls.
Thank you for these waterfalls.

Thank you for my slides and swings.
Thank you for all these things.

If you're worried that your children aren't getting enough daily activity, remember that setting a good example can be very important in changing their behavior. Share with them that you've started a challenging walking program and explain why you've decided it's important to lose some weight and get more physically fit. Encourage your kids to get up off the couch and get moving along with you.

New Walkers Need New Shoes

Your children's feet are still growing, so it's particularly important to find them shoes that fit properly. Ask your pediatrician for advice if you have questions about the type of shoes that are best for your children.

Consider the following advice when buying walking shoes for your children.

- From birth to age 3, your children's feet will grow a half size every three months.
- Shoe size should be re-evaluated every four to six months.

- Don't let them wear hand-me-down shoes—they've already been formed to fit another foot.
- Select from a footwear category based on the function of the shoe. For example, choose from athletic shoes for running and playing, and choose from sturdy supportive shoes for school and everyday walking.
- Don't focus solely on the size. Factor in the overall fit (i.e., length, width, height) of the shoe.
- Don't put toddler socks in socks with "grippers" on the bottom when they're wearing shoes. They inhibit the natural slide of the child's feet in the shoes.

Resources to help you keep your kids healthy

- For help starting a physical activity program for your neighborhood or school, turn to the **President's Council on Physical Fitness** at www.presidents challenge.org.
- Check out the **YMCA's Activate America** program. This program equips the nation's 2,575 YMCAs to become more effective in directly helping individuals and families live healthier lives. Log on to www.ymca.net for more information.
- The **American Red Cross** offers a sports safety training course called "Safe Wheels." The class teaches kindergartners through sixth-graders about basic bicycle safety, including how to prevent bicycle injuries and the importance of helmets. Visit their Web site www.redcross.org for more information.
- Download a free copy of *A Parent's Guide to Healthy Eating and Physical Activity.* This guide contains healthy recipes, money-saving shopping tips, ideas for activities, and much more. For your free copy, go to www.smallstep.gov/sm_steps/news_updates.html.

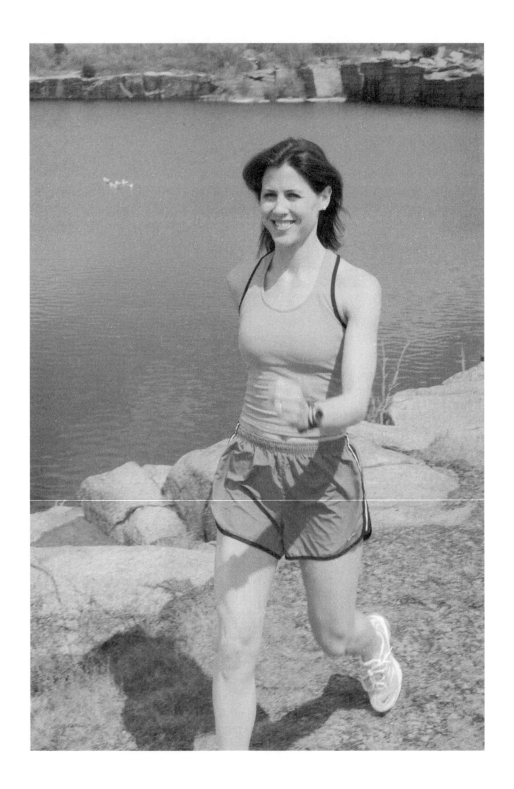

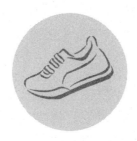

PART THREE

Total Fitness for Guaranteed Weight Loss

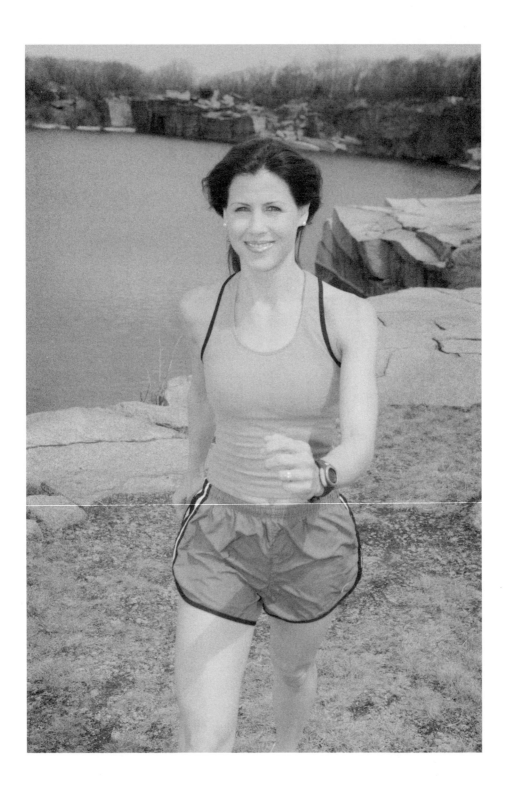

CHAPTER SIX

The Post-Workout Stretching Routine

W E ALL HAVE CRAZY DAYS when finding the time to work out is almost as much of a challenge as doing the workout itself. On those days, we might question whether it's really worth it to take even more precious time to complete some stretches after the walking workout. After all, walking has one of the lowest risks of injury of any exercise, so is stretching really necessary?

In a word, *yes*. Stretching helps keep you flexible, allowing you to retain your full range of motion and easing or preventing any post-workout soreness and tightness. This is especially important when you're doing strenuous workouts such as the ones in this book. Stretching can also improve your balance, and it's a great mental relaxer after a tough workout. In fact, the benefits of stretching extend well beyond your workout to all aspects of your life.

That's why I encourage you to do the stretching routine in this chapter after every workout. (Some of the walking workouts also include specific stretches that target certain additional muscles; when you do those workouts, complete the stretches in this chapter in addition to the workout—specific stretches.)

When doing the following stretches, be careful not to bounce, which can tighten the muscles you're trying to stretch. Stretch until you feel tension, but not so far that you feel pain. And finally, don't rush through the stretches; hold each for the amount of time indicated. The entire sequence will take approximately 13 to 18 minutes to complete.

Because you'll want to give your body a chance to gradually cool down after your workout—and slowly bring your heart rate back down to its normal level—we'll start with the more strenuous standing stretches. Then we'll progress to some less vigorous stretches done while sitting or kneeling, and finally end with a soothing stretch done while lying down that will help relax and center you for the rest of your day.

Calf Stretch on Step: This stretch is great for stretching and lengthening the calf muscles after a strenuous walking workout.

Step both feet up onto a stair or curb. Place your toes at the end of the step, with your heels hanging off the step. If necessary, hold on to a wall or post for support.

Now alternately drop each heel below the level of your toes until you feel a comfortable stretch. Hold for at least 30 seconds. Repeat one or two times with each leg.

Hip Stretch: This stretch is great for walkers as well as for anyone who has to sit most of the day.

Stand tall, with your back straight. Step forward with your right leg, keeping your left foot on the ground. Make sure that your right knee is squarely over the center of your right foot, forming a 90-degree angle.

Tilt your hips forward until you feel a mild stretch in your left hip. Keep your left heel flat. Hold for a slow count of 5. Step back.

Repeat two more times with your right leg forward, then switch legs to stretch your right hip.

Chair Twist: The number one health complaint in America today is back pain. The perfect antidote? This simple stretch that focuses on the lower back.

Sit on the edge of a chair, sideways, with your left side facing the chair back. Throughout the pose, keep your feet and knees together and even. Grasp the back or top of the chair with both hands. Inhale while straightening your spine. As you exhale, twist toward the back of the chair, twisting from the very bottom of your spine, pushing with your left hand and pulling with your right hand. Hold for 30 seconds. Release and switch sides. Repeat one or two times.

Seated Hamstring Stretch: The hamstrings are the muscles that run behind your thighs and knees. Over time, tight, shortened hamstrings can cause shortened stride lengths, so be sure to stretch them out with this targeted move. This stretch is also great for releasing tight muscles in the lower back.

Sit near the edge of a chair, facing a wall. Place your right foot on the floor at the wall, knee straight, and bend your left leg normally. Either place a long towel or a stretching rope (available online or in some sporting goods stores) around the ball of your right foot or hold onto the sides of the chair. Lengthen your back, lift your sternum, and relax your throat, neck, and shoulders. Bend slightly forward from the hip crease, keeping your back elongated. (Be careful not to round your back.) Bend only as far forward as you can with your back straight. Hold for 30 to 45 seconds, then release and switch sides. Repeat once or twice.

Kneeling Hip Stretch: Though it might seem surprising, we store stress in our hips. Perhaps some of the most-used muscles in our bodies are the hip flexors: We depend on them every time we take a step forward. Of course, any time you do any type of exercise, including yoga and Pilates, you're also using your hip flexors. Unfortunately, the hip flexors tend to be one of the tightest muscles in our bodies. Here's a well-deserved stretch for these overworked but dependable muscles.

Kneel on one knee, with your other knee/leg in front of you and your foot flat on the ground in front of you. Keep your upper body straight at all times. Bend at your waist, leaning toward the knee in front of you, until you feel a pull in your hips. Hold for 30 seconds. Switch sides. Repeat one or two times.

Runner's Lunge: It's easy to move from the kneeling stretch into a traditional lunge. The lunge is a little more difficult to do, but when done correctly, it will stretch the quads and calf muscles in addition to the hips.

Stand up and take a large step forward with your right foot, while maintaining a tall, upright upper body. Keep the weight on the heel and mid-foot of the right foot. Next, drop down by bending your left knee, but don't allow it to touch the ground. Hold for 30 seconds, then switch sides. Repeat one or two times.

Modified Downward Facing Dog: This is a traditional yoga move that helps stretch and strengthen your lower back. I've made it easier by using a chair, instead of the floor, as a base.

Place the back of a chair against a wall. Kneel down on both knees 2 to 2½ feet in front of the chair's seat and place your hands on the edge. Come up onto your toes, straighten your legs, lift your buttocks, and angle your torso downward. Work on straightening your arms and legs, lengthening your back as much as possible. Think about moving the front of your thighs toward the back of your thighs. Having a friend pull the top of your thighs back can help you get the full benefit of this pose by taking the weight off your arms. Hold the stretch for 30 seconds. Repeat once or twice.

Note: If this stretch is too easy, you can place your hands either on some thick books you've placed on the floor or directly on the floor instead of on a chair.

Chest Opener: This move opens your lungs for deep breathing and pulls your tight shoulder and chest muscles back.

Roll up a blanket or thick towel. Lie down on the floor with the roll placed under your upper-middle back. If it's more comfortable for you, you can also place a towel or pillow under your head. Close your eyes and relax. Stay in the position as long as you please.

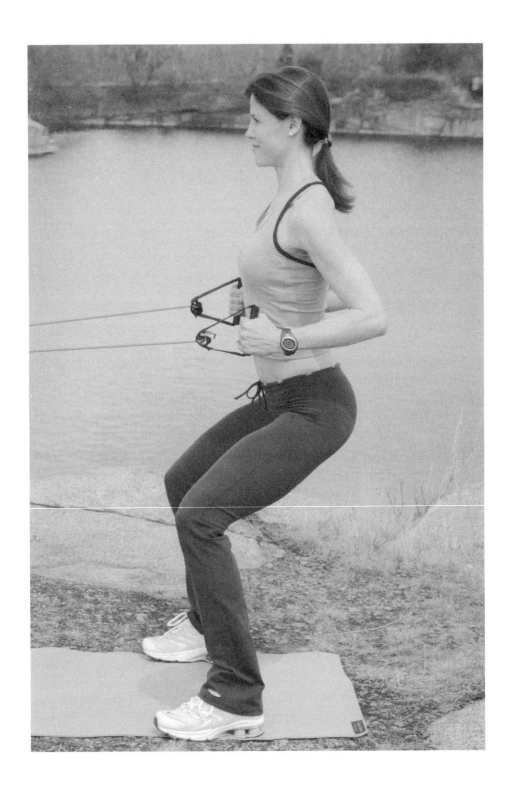

CHAPTER SEVEN

The Strength-Training Workout

To boost your weight-loss efforts, you'll want to combine the walking routines in this book with strength-training moves that build lean muscle. Why? As discussed in chapter 1, muscle is calorie-hungry. A single pound of lean muscle mass requires 35 calories every day just to maintain itself. On the other hand, 1 pound of fat tissue requires only 2 to 3 calories per day. This means that the more muscle you have, the more calories you'll burn, even when you're sleeping or watching TV.

Fortunately, you don't need to get as big as Arnold Schwarzenegger to take advantage of the calorie-burning benefits of lean muscle mass. The exercises in the following strength-training routine won't give you big, bulky muscles; they'll just leave you looking toned and trim. Best of all, they'll give you increased functional strength that will make getting through every part of your day a little easier. Want to know the secret? It's *body weight*.

You see, of all the pieces of exercise equipment that are piled into gyms these days, the one thing that's lacking is floor space. Yet exercises that simply use your own body weight for resistance are quietly becoming the next big thing in the world of physical fitness. Developing functional strength that prepares you for the rigors of your everyday life is more important than completing a fixed-position exercise in a gym. After all, how often are you lying on your back, pressing several pounds away from your chest? Yet that's exactly what the bench press, one of the most popular strength-training moves done in gyms across America, trains you to do. Let's face it: The only time you'd use this move in real life is if you were trapped beneath debris from a hurricane—fortunately, not a likely scenario! The following strength-training workout will tone and prepare your body for the activities you do on a daily basis, things like getting out of bed in the morning, taking the stairs, cooking, cleaning, getting into and out of your car, putting away groceries, and carrying your children or grandchildren around. This is the way to train for weight loss, for functional strength, for life.

Note: Many of my clients have found that doing the following exercises in front of a mirror is extremely helpful (especially when they're using weights). The mirror gives you an additional point of reference as you check for correct body positioning. Not only will you feel what position your body should be in, but you'll be able to see it as well.

Keeping Your Bones Healthy

Many healthy women I know are concerned about osteoporosis, a debilitating disease in which the bones become thinner, more fragile, and more likely to break. Both women and men are at risk for osteoporosis, but women are four times more likely than men to develop the disease. Postmenopausal women are at highest risk for osteoporosis because their bodies produce less estrogen, a key hormone for protecting our bones. A sedentary lifestyle is another risk factor for this disease. Osteoporosis is easy to detect with a bone density test, but it's not so easy to replace lost bone once it's gone or a fracture happens.

One way to maintain healthy bones is to perform weight-bearing exercises such as the ones in the strength-training routine in this chapter. Walking, which is also considered to be a weight-bearing exercise, will also help this condition. In addition, load up on calcium-fortified foods and fluids such as milk, low-fat cheese, yogurt, orange juice, tofu, and broccoli.

Squat

Standing with your legs shoulder-width apart, place all your weight onto your heels. Next, tuck your hips backward and begin to sit down with your arms out in front of you. Maintain your upper-body posture by keeping your eyes focused upward at a 45-degree angle and holding your abdominals in. The bottom point of the movement is established when your knees reach, but do not exceed, 90-degree angles. You'll feel tension in the back of your legs (hamstrings). Next, stand upward, maintaining all other body positions as described for the descent. One repetition should take about 5 seconds (2 seconds descending, 1 second pause, and 2 seconds ascending).

Beginner: Execute the squat as directed above. Aim for 3 sets of 10 to 12 reps each. Concentrate on going through the movement slowly and contracting your lower abdominal muscles, glutes (butt), and hamstring muscles as you lower and lift your body.

Intermediate: Complete 3 sets of 12 to 15 reps each with 3- to 5-pound hand weights held on either side of your hips.

Advanced: Complete 3 sets of 10 to 12 reps each with 8- to 10-pound weights.

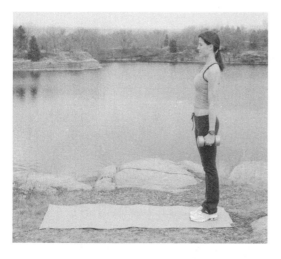

Walking Lunge

Take a large step forward, while maintaining a tall, upright upper body. Strike your lead foot, keeping your weight on the heel and midfoot. Next, drop down by bending your back knee, but don't let it touch the floor. Pause at the bottom and stand back up by lifting your back leg as you travel down your hallway or sidewalk. Your hands and arms can be by your sides, or wherever you feel balanced, but don't place them on your legs for assistance.

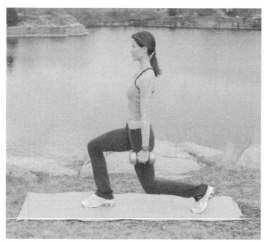

Beginner: Execute the lunge as directed above. Aim for 3 sets of 10 to 12 reps on each leg. Concentrate on going through this movement slowly, keeping your knee right over your toe as your foot lands on the ground for every rep. Push off with your heel as you lift your body back upright.

Intermediate: Complete 3 sets of 12 to 15 reps each while holding a 5-pound medicinc ball.

Advanced: Complete 3 sets of 10 reps each while holding an 8- to 10-pound medicine ball.

Step-Up

Using a staircase, bench, or other platform standing at least 8 inches tall, place one foot up onto the surface and then follow that foot with the second foot. Now you have both feet on the step. Next, step downward with the same foot you began the exercise with, and then step down with the other foot, and repeat.

Beginner: Execute the step-ups as directed above. Aim for a total of 3 sets of 20 reps each (for each set, do 10 reps with your right foot as the lead and 10 with your left foot as the lead for a total of 20 reps). Concentrate on going through this movement slowly, keeping your knee right over your toe as your foot steps up. Push off with your heel as you lift. Try to lower your body off the step "softly" back into your starting position.

Intermediate: Complete 3 sets of 12 to 16 reps (half done with each foot as the lead) while holding 3- to 5-pound hand weights held on either side of your hips. Alternately, hold a 5-pound medicine ball close to your chest as you step up and down.

Advanced: Complete 2 sets of 10 reps each (half done with each foot as the lead), holding 10-pound weights or a 10-pound medicine ball.

Squat Press

Using the same technique as the squat mentioned previously, add a medicine ball, hand weight, or other symmetrically weighted object that you'll hold at your chest with both hands. (I use a medicine ball with handles.) On the downward movement of the squat, keep the medicine ball at your chest. On the ascent portion of the move, begin pressing the ball upward to a position above your head, but remember to keep the ball in your field of peripheral vision. Don't let the ball travel behind your head, as this will place excessive stress on your shoulders and spine. Bring the ball back down to chest level as you descend into the next squat.

Keep your weight evenly distributed on your heels and off your knee joints. If you feel any stress in your lower back, stop the exercise and realign your body, making sure as you begin to sit back that your lower back is not arching.

Beginner: Execute the press with a 1- or 2-pound weight. Aim for 2 sets (rest for 30 seconds between sets) of 10 to 12 presses each.

Intermediate: Complete 2 sets of 12 to 15 reps each with a 5-pound weight.

Advanced: Complete 3 sets of 10 reps each with an 8- to 10-pound weight.

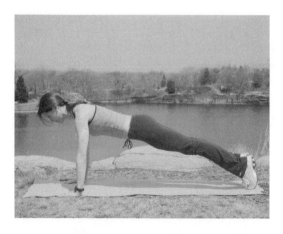

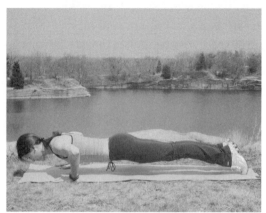

Push-Up

An excellent way to train the chest, arms, and shoulder girdle, the push-up requires no weight except that of your own body. Lying face down, raise your body off the floor with your arms. Your palms should be flat on the floor, spaced shoulder-width apart. Your feet are positioned on their toes, and your body is straight. Keeping your neck in line with your shoulders, gaze about 6 inches in front of you at the floor. Draw your abdominal wall inward to stabilize and support your spine. After setting this position, bend your elbows and lower your body until your torso is 4 to 6 inches from the floor, or you reach a 90-degree angle at your elbow joints. Still maintaining all body positions as previously stated, begin to straighten your arms and raise your body upward. To keep from rushing through each push-up, count to 2 on the descent and then to 2 on the ascent.

Note: Always keep your abdomen pulled up throughout the entire move. Your lower back should not arch. Don't lock your elbows at the top of the movement. For the best results, concentrate on going through the movement slowly.

If you have difficulty completing the move as described above, begin with your knees on the ground, and follow the same movement pattern for the upper body as explained above.

Beginner: Execute the push-up on your knees. Complete 2 sets of 10 reps each, concentrating on going through the movement slowly.

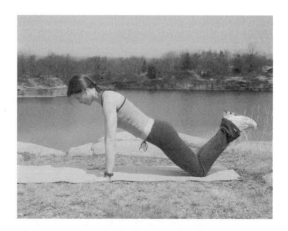

Intermediate: Complete 3 sets of 12 to 15 reps each. Do 2 sets on your toes and 1 set on your knees. Rest for 10 to 15 seconds in a yoga Child's Pose between sets.

To complete the Child's Pose: Kneel on the floor. Sit on your heels and separate your knees as wide as your hips. Lay your torso down between your thighs. Lift the base of your skull away from the back of your neck and lay your hands on the floor by your torso. Turn your palms up and relax your shoulders toward the floor. To come up, first lengthen your torso, then lift your back up—sitting with your lower legs under you—again on your heels. Reach your hands out in front of you, push up onto your toes, and pull your abs in—now you're back into a push-up position.

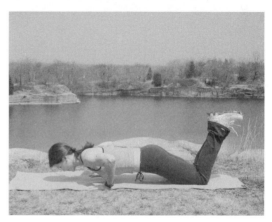

Advanced: Complete 3 sets of 12 to 15 reps each, all on your toes. Rest for 10 to 15 seconds in a yoga Child's Pose between sets.

Hip Lift

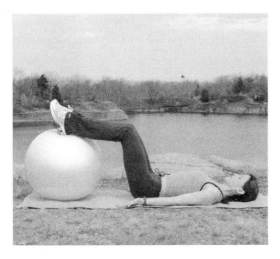

Lie on your back on the floor, with your legs slightly flexed and positioned atop a physioball. Press your heels into the north pole of the ball. Next, press into the ball with your legs, raising your torso off the floor. Lift your hips until you can't raise them any further. Your arms should be by your sides, palms up, at all times, and your head, neck, and shoulders relaxed and against the floor. Hold this position for 3 to 5 seconds while you tuck and lift, then release.

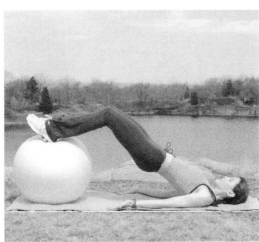

If you have difficulty performing this exercise, use the floor as your base of support, instead of the physioball. After you feel comfortable, you can then advance to using the physioball.

Beginner: Complete 10 reps, performing them without the ball, if necessary.

Intermediate: Complete 15 reps.

Advanced: Complete 20 reps.

Single-Leg Hip Lift

Get into the same position as above, but this time, elevate one leg toward the ceiling. This position is very difficult and should be attempted only after the dual-leg hip lift is mastered. Hold this position for 3 to 5 seconds while you tuck and lift, then release.

Beginner: Complete 10 reps (5 with each leg elevated).

Intermediate: Complete 20 reps (10 with each leg elevated).

Advanced: Complete 30 reps (15 with each leg elevated).

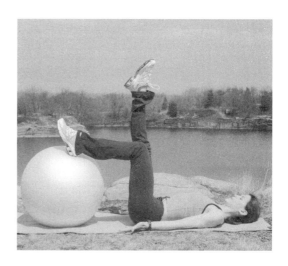

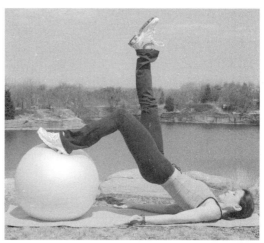

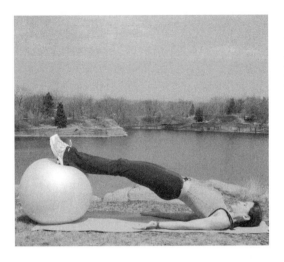

Hamstring Curl

Use the same set-up position as the hip lift. As you reach the top position of the lift, begin to curl your legs beneath your thighs, bringing your heels inward as far as you comfortably can without compromising your body position. It's very important to keep the full hip lift while curling in. The hamstrings perform two functions: hip extension and knee flexion. Completing both tasks simultaneously will maximize hamstring work. Repeat the curl.

Beginner: Complete 2 sets of 10 reps each.

Intermediate: Complete 3 sets of 10 reps each.

Advanced: Complete 3 sets of 15 reps each.

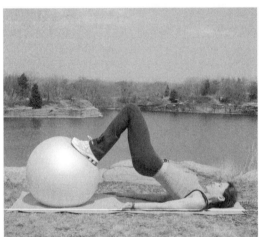

Single-Leg Hamstring Curl

Get into the same position as above, but this time, keep one leg on the ball and raise the other leg toward the ceiling. This move is very difficult, and should be performed only if you've mastered the hamstring curl and hip lift.

Beginner: Complete 1 set of 10 reps for each leg.

Intermediate: Complete 2 sets of 12 reps each for each leg.

Advanced: 2 sets of 15 to 18 reps each for each leg.

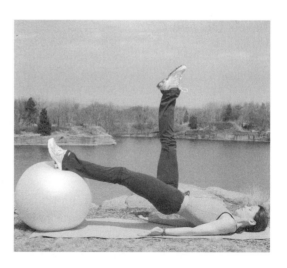

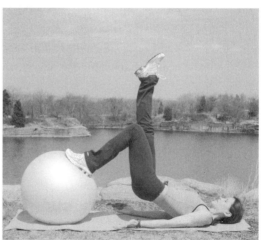

Biceps Curl

Grasp both handles of an exercise band with your palms facing forward and step on the loop portion of the band. Your legs and hands should be shoulder-width apart. Flexing your knees slightly, and keeping your torso tall and your abs tight, with your eyes forward and your chin up, curl the handles toward the front of your shoulders. Stop the movement when your hands are 90 degrees from your shoulder. Be sure to keep your elbows close to your torso throughout the entire movement. Pause for a brief moment at the top, then slowly descend, stopping the motion just before your elbows are straight.

Alternately, you can complete the biceps curls with hand weights instead of the exercise band. Use enough weight that you can complete only the desired number of reps; the last one should be difficult, but not impossible. If you find you're swinging the weight to get it up, lower the weight and slow down. Also, remember not to touch your shoulders when you lift the weight; keep your elbows from moving back and forth.

Beginner: Complete 1 set of 14 to 16 reps using a 3-pound weight or an exercise band that is challenging but allows you to complete each set.

Intermediate: Complete 3 sets of 8 to 10 reps each using a 5- to 8-pound weight or an exercise band that is challenging but allows you to complete each set.

Advanced: Complete 3 sets of 10 to 16 reps each using a 8- to 10-pound weight or an exercise band that is challenging but allows you to complete each set.

Physioball Ab Crunch

The physioball is a great tool for strengthening the abs, or *rectus abdominis,* muscles. Lie face-up with the ball resting under your mid/lower back. Place your feet firmly on the floor about 2 feet in front of you and shoulder-width apart. Cross your arms over your chest or place them behind the base of your head. Contract your abs to lift your torso off the ball, pulling the bottom of your rib cage down toward your hips. When you curl up, keep the ball still (don't roll). As you lower back down, you should feel a stretch in your abs without an arch in your lower back.

Beginner: Complete 1 set of 10 reps.

Intermediate: Complete 2 sets of 12 to 15 reps each.

Advanced: Complete 3 sets of 15 to 20 reps each.

Squat-Row

Wrap your exercise band around a pole or the leg of a bench. Then grasp both handles of the band, with your palms facing each other. Your stance will mimic that of the squat position discussed earlier. Reach your arms straight out in front of you. Begin your descent into the squat, keeping your arms at shoulder level and still straight forward. Next, as you begin to rise from the bottom of the squat, begin to pull the band using a rowing motion. Once your hands nearly reach your chest, pause for a brief moment as you should also have reached the top of the squat. Now standing and holding the tubing taut, begin to descend, while slowing releasing the row back toward its original position. Repeat.

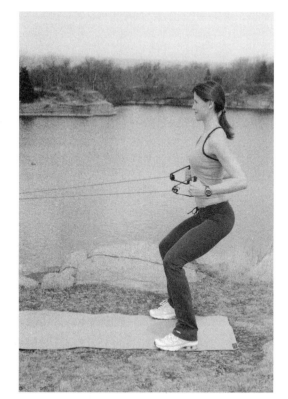

Beginner: Complete 1 set of 12 reps.

Intermediate: Complete 2 sets of 12 to 15 reps.

Advanced: Complete 3 sets of 12 to 15 reps.

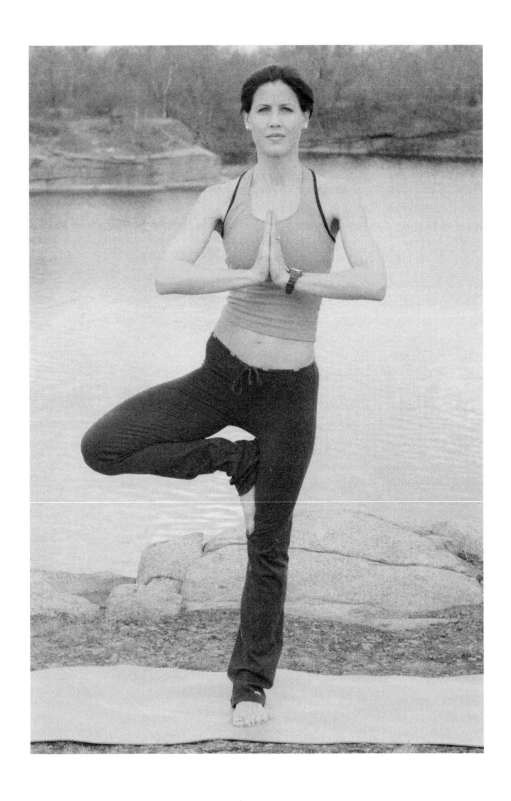

CHAPTER EIGHT

The Yoga and Pilates Routine

YOGA AND PILATES ARE TWO OF THE MOST POPULAR EXERCISE REGIMENS in the fitness world today—and for good reason. Both of these practices offer low-impact but challenging workouts based on the understanding that flexibility and core strength are major components of physical fitness. Increasing your flexibility and core strength improves your range of motion, overall strength, posture, and mental well-being and health.

The practice of yoga, more so than Pilates, is rooted in spiritual health combining self-awareness, deep breathing, and inner healing. Pilates, on the other hand, is a slightly more physically active approach. It adds the component of strength training with a series of machines, mat work, and often the use of a physioball. Both disciplines require you to create a portion or whole part of the exercise movement by bringing your body into a set position unregulated by a machine. Pilates has a stronger focus on the self-recruitment of the abdominal muscles, a move that becomes the starting and focal point of each Pilates exercise.

Yoga

Yoga is good for what ails you. Specifically, research shows that yoga helps manage or control conditions as diverse as anxiety, arthritis, asthma, back pain, blood pressure, carpal tunnel syndrome, chronic fatigue, depression, diabetes, epilepsy, headaches, heart disease, and multiple sclerosis. What's more, yoga:

- Reduces stress and tension
- Boosts self-esteem
- Improves circulation

- Stimulates the immune system

- Creates a sense of well-being and calm

Developed in India, yoga is a spiritual practice that has been evolving over the past 5,000 years. The original yogis were reacting, in part, to India's ancient Vedic religion, which emphasized rituals. The yogis wanted a direct spiritual experience—one on one—not symbolic ritual. So they developed yoga. In Sanskrit, the classical language of India, yoga means "union."

According to the yogis, true happiness, liberation, and enlightenment comes from union with the divine consciousness, known as Brahman, or with Atman, the transcendent Self. The various yoga practices are a methodology for reaching that goal. There are several different types of yoga. In hatha yoga, for example, postures and breathing exercises help purify the mind, body, and spirit so the yogi can attain union. I recommend trying out a number of different yoga practices to find the one that best fits your lifestyle.

Our Posture Matters

The essence of good posture is a natural skeletal balance maintained by muscles strong enough to hold everything in place. In fact, it's almost impossible to have good posture and *not* be fit. Our back and abdominal muscles must be strong and flexible to support our spines, so strengthening and stretching are key. Pilates, yoga, tai chi, and other movements that exercise your core will help. But you also have to do some homework away from your workouts.

Sit up tall, not slouched, in front of the computer, TV, and steering wheel. Also, try doing a few shoulder rolls throughout the day to ease any tension in your shoulders and back. (Simply stand or sit with your feet shoulder-width apart, and then slowly roll your shoulders forward. After doing this a few times, roll your shoulders slowly backward.) My husband, Chris, occasionally sits in front of his desk on a stability ball. Sitting on this unstable surface forces your body to recruit your abdominal muscles to help you sit up straight.

To learn more about the benefits of good posture, visit www.postureguide.com.

In yoga, pranayama breathing exercises help clear the *nadis,* or channels, that carry *prana,* the universal life force, allowing it to flow freely. Yogis believe that when the channels are clear and the last block at the base of the spine has been opened, a potent spiritual energy called Kundalini rises through the spine, through the central channel called the sushumna-nadi, and joins the crown chakra. (Sanskrit for "wheel" or disk," *chakra* refers to a basic energy center in the body. In these traditions, there are seven basic chakras, and they all exist within the subtle body, overlaying the physical body. Through modern physiology we can see that these seven chakras correspond exactly to the seven main nerve ganglia that emanate from the spinal column.) According to yogi tradition, the release of Kundalini leads to enlightenment and union.

Pilates

Though Pilates is a much newer discipline, it is a wonderful complement to yoga. This exercise regimen was developed by Joseph Pilates (1880–1967), whose frailty as a child—he suffered from rickets, asthma, and rheumatic fever-sparked his intense interest in and study of anatomy and various forms of exercise. He grew to become an accomplished gymnast, boxer, skier, and diver. The exercise discipline he created focuses on improving flexibility and strength without building bulk. It offers a great way to build lean, long muscles and a strong core.

I had the pleasure of meeting Joseph and his wife, Clara, many years ago. I found them both to be true inspirations! They put me through my paces on the Reformer pulley machine, a piece of Pilates equipment that Joseph designed.

Today, Pilates exercises are used by individuals as well as dance companies, sports teams, and even members of Broadway shows. If you'd like to try out a Pilates class, check your local gym or YMCA. Because of its popularity, classes in Pilates usually aren't hard to find. Be aware, however, that because Joseph Pilates didn't patent his exercises, there are now many forms of "pilates" in existence. I recommend that you stick with classes taught by instructors who are certified with the American College of Sports Medicine.

Pilates incorporates the following guidelines, which make up the foundation of the Pilates technique.

Breathe. Pilates incorporates a kind of breathing called "bellows action," expanding the ribs sideways like an accordion to fill the lungs.

Energize. Oxygenated blood is forced into the farthest reaches of the body, flushing out toxins in what Joseph Pilates called an "internal shower."

Align. Proper alignment is essential. Focus is placed on neutralizing the spine and maintaining its natural curvature. Also, each movement is initiated from the core by precisely engaging the abdominal muscles.

Move. Regular Pilates workouts produce heightened body awareness and control that become an integrated part of the everyday movements of a person's life.

The Program

The following routine is a collection of my favorite yoga and Pilates moves. These poses are biomechanically sound, effective, and safe. They offer a perfect complement to the advanced walking workouts in part two of the book, challenging your muscles in new ways that strengthen them even further. If you'd like, you can perform the following moves on a mat. Otherwise, simply do them on a soft, carpeted floor.

If you find this routine enjoyable and would like to practice additional yoga and Pilates positions, visit www.yogabasics.com.

There are controversial moves in both yoga and Pilates. Here's some good advice for you: No matter what your physical condition, avoid any exercise move or class that is preceded with a caution, such as "If you have back problems or pain, don't do this exercise." My professional opinion is that if it's problematic enough to aggravate an existing condition, it also has the ability to start one.

Table

In addition to starting the routine with this position, you'll be returning to this neutral position in between the other poses in the following routine. To get in Table position, get on the floor on your hands and knees, with your feet behind you and your spine in a neutral position. Look at the floor directly in front of your hands.

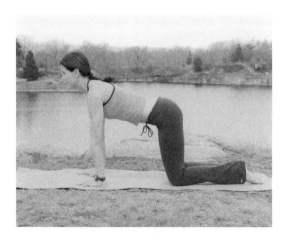

Downward Facing Dog

Stretches the hamstrings, lower back, and calves.

From the Table position, tuck your toes under and lift your hips up toward the ceiling. Spread your fingers wide apart with the middle finger facing forward and the palms shoulder-width apart. Press your fingers and palms into the floor.

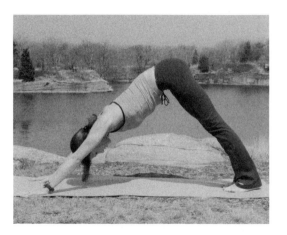

Using straight arms, press your hips up and back. Keep your spine straight and long. Your feet should be hip-width apart and your toes facing forward. Press your heels into the floor until you feel a stretch in the back of your legs. Your legs should either be straight, or slightly bent at the knees to keep your back flat.

Let your head and neck hang freely from your shoulders or look up at your belly button. Breathe and hold for 2 to 6 breaths.

To release: Bend your knees and lower your hips back to Table position.

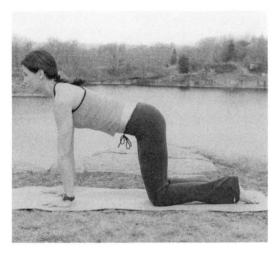

Cat Pose

Stretches the middle to upper back and shoulders.

From Table pose, exhale and tuck your tailbone under, round your spine, and let your head drop down. Press into your palms to drop your shoulders away from your ears and to reach your middle and upper back up toward the ceiling. Breathe and hold for 4 to 8 breaths.

To release: Inhale and flatten your back to move into Table pose.

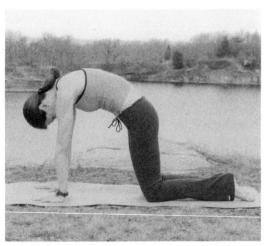

Modified Bridge

Builds core and lower-body strength, lengthens and strengthens the spine, energizes the body, and stimulates the endocrine and nervous systems.

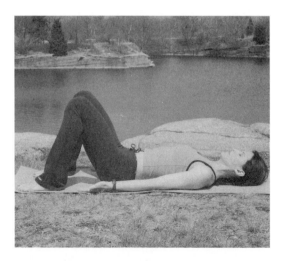

Lying on your back, bend both knees and place your feet flat on the floor, hip-width apart. Slide your arms alongside your body with your palms facing up. Your fingertips should be lightly touching your heels.

Press your feet into the floor, inhale, and lift your hips up, rolling your spine off the floor. Lightly squeeze your knees together to keep them hip-width apart.

Press down into your arms and shoulders to lift your chest up. Engage your legs and buttocks to lift your hips higher. Breathe and hold for 4 to 8 breaths.

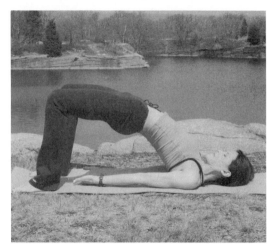

To release: Exhale and slowly roll your spine back to the floor.

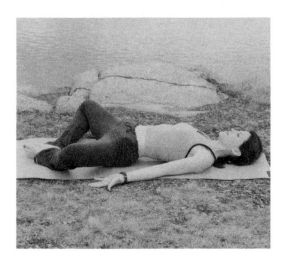

Reclining Angle Pose

Stretches the muscles we use every time we walk, including inner thighs, hip flexors, and groin muscles. This pose can be modified to meet any level of resistance in the hips and groin.

Lying on your back, put the soles of your feet together and pull your legs as close to your pelvis as is comfortable. Press your outer thighs away from the sides of your torso, releasing your lower back, torso, and buttocks toward the floor.

Lay your arms on the floor, angled at about 45 degrees from the sides of your torso, palms up. As your groins drop toward the floor, so will your knees.

If you feel any strain in the inner thighs or groin, try to modify by supporting your thighs on a block or folded blanket. Breathe and hold for 4 to 8 breaths.

To release: Exhale and gently release the arms and legs.

Child's Pose

Gently stretches the lower back, massages and tones the abdominal organs, and stimulates digestion and elimination.

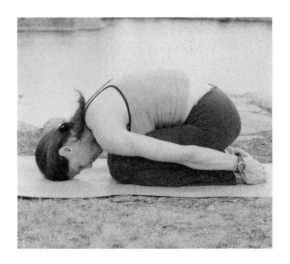

From a kneeling position, sit on your heels and slowly lower your chest down toward your thighs. Rest your head, arms, and hips down toward the floor. (If your head doesn't quite reach the floor, place a pillow between your forehead and the floor.)

Try to reach your sitting bones towards your heels. Breathe and hold for 4 to 12 breaths.

To release: Place palms under the shoulders and slowly inhale up to a seated position.

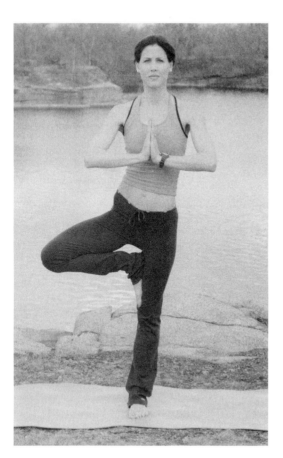

Tree Pose

Improves our balance, strengthens our thighs, calves, ankles, feet and "core" (abs and back); also increases the flexibility of our hips and groin.

Lift one leg up placing the sole of your foot either on your shin or inner thigh (above or below your knee), toes pointing down. Once you are steady, float your hands towards your heart. If you can't get steady, use a wall or a high-back chair for support. Breathe and hold for 4 to 8 breaths. Repeat with your other leg. A variation would be to bring your arms overhead and join your palms together.

To release: Slowly exhale your arms down and release your legs.

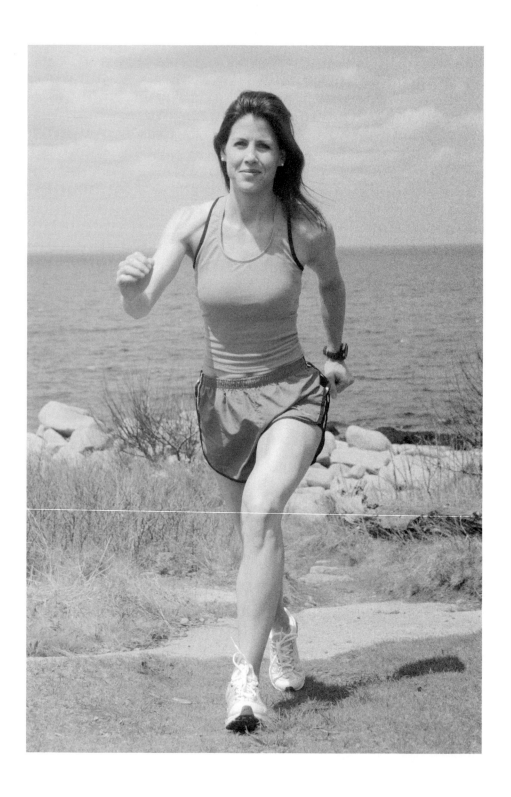

Walking Logs

USE THE FOLLOWING LOGS to keep track of your daily progress. As the weeks pass, refer back to your earlier logs to see just how far you've come (both in terms of miles and strength!). I've provided a week's worth of logs here; simply photocopy these pages as needed. I recommend keeping them all together in a three-ring binder. If you don't have access to a copier, you can also simply jot down the information in a notebook and keep your log that way. Whichever way you choose, taking the few minutes each day to fill in your log will be time well spent.

Remember, also, that maintaining a healthy weight requires a dedication to remaining active every day, even when you're not scheduled to complete a walking workout. That's why I recommend wearing a pedometer, especially on days you're scheduled only to do the strength-training routine. This way, you can make sure you're staying active throughout the day by monitoring the number of steps you take.

Today's Date: _____ **Workout Month #** _____ **Workout Week #** _____

Monday

Name of Walking Workout You Completed: _____

Level Completed (circle one): *Beginner* *Intermediate* *Advanced*

If you didn't complete the workout as described in part two (for example, you didn't complete the full number of recommended strength-training reps or you walked for a longer or shorter amount of time), write down what you did complete here:

_____

_____

_____

Did you complete the Post-Workout Stretching Routine?   YES   NO

If directed to do so, did you complete the Yoga and Pilates Routine?   YES   NO

If you were scheduled to complete the Strength-Training
Routine today, did you?   YES   NO

If yes, which level of the Strength-Training Routine did you complete (circle one)?
Beginner *Intermediate* *Advanced*

Now take a few moments to write down how you felt before, during, and after your workout.

_____

_____

_____

Pedometer Check: If you didn't have a scheduled walking workout today, how many steps did you take from morning to bedtime? _____

Was there anything that got in the way of your workout today? If so, what can you do to resolve it so that your exercise program doesn't get derailed?

_____

_____

Today's Date: _____   Workout Month # _____   Workout Week #_____

Tuesday

Name of Walking Workout You Completed: _____

Level Completed (circle one):   *Beginner   Intermediate   Advanced*

If you didn't complete the workout as described in part two (for example, you didn't complete the full number of recommended strength-training reps or you walked for a longer or shorter amount of time), write down what you did complete here:

_____

_____

_____

Did you complete the Post-Workout Stretching Routine?   YES   NO

If directed to do so, did you complete the Yoga and Pilates Routine?   YES   NO

If you were scheduled to complete the Strength-Training
Routine today, did you?   YES   NO

If yes, which level of the Strength-Training Routine did you complete (circle one)?
Beginner   Intermediate   Advanced

Now take a few moments to write down how you felt before, during, and after your workout.

_____

_____

_____

Pedometer Check: If you didn't have a scheduled walking workout today, how many steps did you take from morning to bedtime? _____

Was there anything that got in the way of your workout today? If so, what can you do to resolve it so that your exercise program doesn't get derailed?

_____

_____

Today's Date: _____ **Workout Month #** _____ **Workout Week #** _____

Wednesday

Name of Walking Workout You Completed: _____

Level Completed (circle one): *Beginner   Intermediate   Advanced*

If you didn't complete the workout as described in part two (for example, you didn't complete the full number of recommended strength-training reps or you walked for a longer or shorter amount of time), write down what you did complete here:

_____

_____

_____

Did you complete the Post-Workout Stretching Routine?   YES   NO

If directed to do so, did you complete the Yoga and Pilates Routine?   YES   NO

If you were scheduled to complete the Strength-Training
Routine today, did you?   YES   NO

If yes, which level of the Strength-Training Routine did you complete (circle one)?
Beginner   Intermediate   Advanced

Now take a few moments to write down how you felt before, during, and after your workout.

_____

_____

_____

Pedometer Check: If you didn't have a scheduled walking workout today, how many steps did you take from morning to bedtime? _____

Was there anything that got in the way of your workout today? If so, what can you do to resolve it so that your exercise program doesn't get derailed?

_____

_____

Today's Date: _____ Workout Month # _____ Workout Week #_____

Thursday

Name of Walking Workout You Completed: _____

Level Completed (circle one): *Beginner* *Intermediate* *Advanced*

If you didn't complete the workout as described in part two (for example, you didn't complete the full number of recommended strength-training reps or you walked for a longer or shorter amount of time), write down what you did complete here:

_____

_____

_____

Did you complete the Post-Workout Stretching Routine?   YES   NO

If directed to do so, did you complete the Yoga and Pilates Routine?   YES   NO

If you were scheduled to complete the Strength-Training
Routine today, did you?   YES   NO

If yes, which level of the Strength-Training Routine did you complete (circle one)?
Beginner   *Intermediate*   *Advanced*

Now take a few moments to write down how you felt before, during, and after your workout.

_____

_____

_____

Pedometer Check: If you didn't have a scheduled walking workout today, how many steps did you take from morning to bedtime? _____

Was there anything that got in the way of your workout today? If so, what can you do to resolve it so that your exercise program doesn't get derailed?

_____

_____

Today's Date: ______ **Workout Month #** ______ **Workout Week #**______

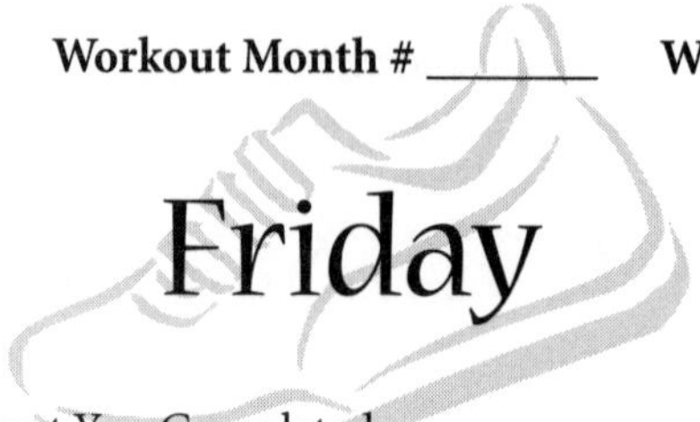

Friday

Name of Walking Workout You Completed: ______________________________

Level Completed (circle one): *Beginner* *Intermediate* *Advanced*

If you didn't complete the workout as described in part two (for example, you didn't complete the full number of recommended strength-training reps or you walked for a longer or shorter amount of time), write down what you did complete here:

____

____

____

Did you complete the Post-Workout Stretching Routine? YES NO

If directed to do so, did you complete the Yoga and Pilates Routine? YES NO

If you were scheduled to complete the Strength-Training Routine today, did you? YES NO

If yes, which level of the Strength-Training Routine did you complete (circle one)?
Beginner *Intermediate* *Advanced*

Now take a few moments to write down how you felt before, during, and after your workout.

____

____

____

Pedometer Check: If you didn't have a scheduled walking workout today, how many steps did you take from morning to bedtime? _________

Was there anything that got in the way of your workout today? If so, what can you do to resolve it so that your exercise program doesn't get derailed?

____

____

Today's Date: _____   Workout Month # _____   Workout Week #_____

Saturday

Name of Walking Workout You Completed: _____

Level Completed (circle one):   *Beginner   Intermediate   Advanced*

If you didn't complete the workout as described in part two (for example, you didn't complete the full number of recommended strength-training reps or you walked for a longer or shorter amount of time), write down what you did complete here:

_____

_____

_____

Did you complete the Post-Workout Stretching Routine?   YES   NO

If directed to do so, did you complete the Yoga and Pilates Routine?   YES   NO

If you were scheduled to complete the Strength-Training
Routine today, did you?   YES   NO

If yes, which level of the Strength-Training Routine did you complete (circle one)?
Beginner   Intermediate   Advanced

Now take a few moments to write down how you felt before, during, and after your workout.

_____

_____

_____

Pedometer Check: If you didn't have a scheduled walking workout today, how many steps did you take from morning to bedtime? _____

Was there anything that got in the way of your workout today? If so, what can you do to resolve it so that your exercise program doesn't get derailed?

_____

_____

Today's Date: _____ **Workout Month #** _____ **Workout Week #** _____

Sunday

Name of Walking Workout You Completed: _____

Level Completed (circle one): *Beginner* *Intermediate* *Advanced*

If you didn't complete the workout as described in part two (for example, you didn't complete the full number of recommended strength-training reps or you walked for a longer or shorter amount of time), write down what you did complete here:

_____

_____

_____

Did you complete the Post-Workout Stretching Routine?   YES   NO

If directed to do so, did you complete the Yoga and Pilates Routine?   YES   NO

If you were scheduled to complete the Strength-Training
Routine today, did you?   YES   NO

If yes, which level of the Strength-Training Routine did you complete (circle one)?
Beginner   *Intermediate*   *Advanced*

Now take a few moments to write down how you felt before, during, and after your workout.

_____

_____

_____

Pedometer Check: If you didn't have a scheduled walking workout today, how many steps did you take from morning to bedtime? _____

Was there anything that got in the way of your workout today? If so, what can you do to resolve it so that your exercise program doesn't get derailed?

_____

_____

Glossary

Aerobic exercise: Sustained, repetitive work that strengthens the heart and lungs and increases the body's metabolism. Types of aerobic exercise include walking, running, cycling, and swimming.

Anaerobic exercise: Literally meaning "without oxygen," anaerobic exercises are short and intense. During anaerobic exercise, the muscles being used don't have the benefit of extra oxygen. Anaerobic exercises build up muscle and make your body mass leaner, which means you can burn more calories even while at rest. Perhaps the best-known form of anaerobic exercise is resistance training.

Body mass index (BMI): This is a calculation that uses your height and weight to estimate how much body fat you have. Too much body fat is a problem because it can lead to illnesses and other health problems. BMI is a good but not perfect method for judging how much body fat someone has because a more muscular person may have a higher weight and BMI but not much body fat. Also, a smaller-framed person could have an ideal BMI, but might have less muscle and too much body fat.

Chakra: In yoga tradition, *chakra* refers to a basic energy center in the body.

Coolmax: A "hydrophobic" (water-hating) polyester fabric with fiber cross sections that produce a strong wicking action; often used in outerwear linings and light layering garments. Manufactured by INVISTA.

Kundalini: A potent spiritual energy that, yogis believe, lies dormant at the base of the spine but can be released through special breathing exercises. According to yogic tradition, the release of kundalini leads to enlightenment and union.

Last: The mold on which shoes are formed. There are three types of lasts: straight, semi-curved, and curved.

Maximum Heart Rate: The greatest number of times per minute the heart is capable of beating. Your maximum heart rate is determined by subtracting your age from 220. Never work out at your maximum heart rate.

Metabolism: All of the processes that occur in the body that turn the food you eat into energy your body can use.

Midsole: The part of a shoe located between the outer sole, which touches the ground, and the shoe upper.

Overpronation: An excessive inward roll of the foot after landing (see *pronation*). Overpronation causes stress first on the plantar fascia and then upward to the knees and hips. In particular, people with flat feet can be at risk for overpronation. A sign of overpronation is excessive wear on the inner soles of the shoes.

Perceived Exertion (PE): A method for determining how hard you're working by monitoring how difficult the exercise feels as you're doing it. When you measure your PE, you need to pay special attention to factors such as how hard you're breathing, how much you're sweating, and how tired your muscles feel. Benefits of using PE include the ability to monitor your exercise intensity without equipment and without having to stop to "check" it, as is necessary with heart-rate monitoring.

Physioball: A large ball made of heavy-duty rubber, a physioball is used for developing strength, flexibility, and balance. It's also known as a Swiss, fitness, or stability ball.

Pilates: An exercise regimen developed by Joseph Pilates that focuses on improving flexibility and strength. Most Pilates programs include strength training with a series of machines, mat work, and sometimes the use of a physioball.

Plantar fascia: The broad band of fibrous tissue that runs along the bottom of the foot.

Pronation: The natural inward "rolling," or rotating, of the sole of the foot (particularly the heel and arch) that occurs during the heel strike portion of the step.

Rep: One completed exercise. Short for "repetition."

Resistance training: Another name for strength training, this type of exercise uses weight or resistance to tone muscle.

Set: A series of completed repetitions done with little or no pause between them.

Shin splints: Term for the pain felt on the front and inside of the lower leg due to inflamed muscles and/or tendons.

Strength training: Any exercise that uses weight or resistance to tone muscle. This may include free weights, such as dumbbells; stationary weights, such as the weight machines found in most gyms; resistance bands; medicine balls; or the body's own weight, such as in a push-up.

Target heart rate zone: A safe but effective range in which your heart rate should fall while you're exercising.

Toe box: The part of a shoe that encases the toes.

Underpronation: Also known as supination, underpronation occurs when the feet don't roll inward enough after landing (see *pronation*). Underpronation may occur when a walker is wearing the wrong style of shoe for his foot shape and can lead to painful shins and joints, or even injury.

Yoga: Literally meaning "union," yoga combines self-awareness and inner healing. Originating in India, the practice of yoga is believed to be more than 5,000 years old. While there are many types of yoga, perhaps the most famous is hatha yoga, which is a complex system of postures and breathing exercises that help to keep the body strong and supple and aid you in drawing your attention inward.

Resources

I suggest these organizations, Web sites, and manufacturers to go to for more information.

General Information on Walking and Physical Fitness

National Organization of Mall Walkers: Some 2,400 malls nationwide let walkers in before shopping hours. Many have walking clubs. Contact the National Organization of Mall Walkers at PO Box 191, Hermann, MO 65041 to find the club nearest you.

The Pilates Physical Mind Institute: You can find general Pilates information as well as information on Pilates certification, equipment, and even a studio finder at www.the-method.com.

The President's Council on Physical Fitness and Sports: This committee of volunteer citizens not only advises the President (through the Secretary of Health and Human Services) about physical activity, fitness, and sports in America, but it also acts as a catalyst to promote health and physical fitness to people of all ages and backgrounds. Visit the Council's Web site at www.fitness.gov to learn about the Council and its work and for links to other fitness-oriented government and private Web sites. You can also contact the Council by calling (202) 690-9000 or writing to President's Council on Physical Fitness and Sports, Department W, 200 Independence Avenue SW, Room 738-H, Washington, D.C., 20201-0004.

Racewalk.com: This Web site gives you all the information you need to learn to race walk. It also provides information on upcoming race-walking events and race-walking clubs in your area.

WalkSport: This organization manages many mall-walking programs in various malls across the country. For a small yearly fee, the organization provides a plastic card that you swipe through an electronic reader before and after you walk at participating malls. For every 50 hours you walk, you'll receive a certificate redeemable for special prizes. To learn more about the program, visit www.walksport.com, call (800) 757-WALK (9255), or write to WalkSport, 9280 South Kyrene Road, Suite 134, Tempe, AZ 85284.

Yoga Basics: Visit www.yogabasics.com for detailed information on numerous yoga poses as well as the benefits and history of yoga.

Recommended Fitness Equipment Manufacturers

Though this list is not exclusive, the following companies make products I have used and recommend.

Baby Walking and Jogging Strollers: Visit both www.gracobaby.com and www.bobgear.com to find out about the latest in strollers that also allow you to get a great workout.

NordicTrack: Visit www.nordictrack.com for information on their ViewPoint Treadmill and www.inclinetrainer.com for information on the Incline TrainerX10.

Perform Better: This company sells a wide variety of exercise bands. Visit www.performbetter.com or call (888) 556-7464.

Polar Electro Inc.: Makers of the Polar Heart Rate Monitor, this company can be found online at www.polarusa.com. Or call (800) 227-1314.

Resist-A-Ball: This manufacturer of physioballs can be reached at www.resista-ball.com or (877) 269-9893.

SmartWool: This company offers wool socks, long underwear, and other garments that are specially designed not to shrink or cause itching. Visit www.smartwool.com or call (800) 550-WOOL (9665).

True Fitness Treadmills: This company's treadmills are constructed with special-grade shock-absorbing treads, which offer you greater cushioning as you walk. Visit www.truefitness.com or call (800) 426-6570.

Xvest: A weighted vest to try is the XVest. Their Web site is www.thexvest.com.

Information on Walking and Hiking Vacations

American Discovery Trail: Visit www.discoverytrail.org to learn more about this amazing recreational trail that stretches across the United States. Running through 15 states, it stretches for more than 6,800 nonmotorized miles. The Web site offers a state-by-state trail directory, so you can head out for an afternoon walk or venture out on a multiple-day journey.

Backroads: Visit www.backroads.com to request a catalog of this company's biking, walking, or hiking vacations. Or call (800) GO-ACTIVE (462-2848).

The Walking Connection: This company offers walking and hiking vacations in locales throughout the world. Their Web site offers information on fitness walking as well as links to other walking sites. You can also sign up for two free e-newsletters. Visit www.walkingconnection.com or call (800) 295-WALK (9255).

Recommended Reading

Books

American Dietetic Association Complete Food and Nutrition Guide by Roberta Larson Duyff. Wiley, 2002. A comprehensive guide to eating well, with nutritional advice for every stage of life.

Asanas: 608 Yoga Poses by Dharma Mittra. New World Library, 2003. This book offers helpful visual descriptions of each yoga pose.

Encyclopedia of Sports and Fitness Nutrition by Liz Applegate. Prima Lifestyles, 2002. Shows you how to develop a nutrition plan that will help you to get the most out of your workouts.

Healing Moves by Carol Krucoff and Mitchell Krucoff, MD. Three Rivers Press, 2001.

Healthy Kids: Help Them Eat Smart and Stay Active—For Life! by Marilu Henner. Regan Books, 2004. This book offers lots of recipes for meals and snacks the whole family will enjoy.

Mediterranean Diet Cookbook : A Delicious Alternative for Lifelong Health by Nancy Jenkins. Bantam, 1994. Offers delicious, healthful recipes based on the Mediterranean diet.

The South Beach Diet: The Delicious, Doctor-Designed, Foolproof Plan for Fast and Healthy Weight Loss by Arthur Agatston. Rodale, 2003. This book gives readers some concrete strategies for eating a balanced diet.

Strength Training Anatomy by Frédéric Delavier. Human Kinetics Publishers, 2001. This book provides an inside view of muscles in action.

The Whartons' Stretch Book: Active-Isolated Stretching by Jim and Phil Wharton. Three Rivers Press, 1996. This book includes a 20-minute stretching routine that is divided into five body zones.

Magazines

Cooking Light: This magazine offers delicious, light recipes, plus information on exercise and maintaining a healthy lifestyle. To learn more or place a subscription, visit www.cookinglight.com.

Men's Journal: Visit www.mensjournal.com. This magazine is not just for men. The editors offer lots of great fitness tips, information about working out in the great outdoors, and inspirational stories about athletes.

Natural Health: To maintain good health and fitness, we need to know the facts about the foods we eat. This magazine offers helpful information on natural and alternative products for adults and children. Their Web site is www.naturalhealthmag.com.

Outside: To order a subscription or read their online content, visit www.outside.away.com. If you need inspiration to hit the hills, trails, or even sidewalks around your house, this is the magazine to read. The editors do the research and live the outdoors lifestyle. I've passed a couple of them on the hiking trails in Santa Fe, New Mexico, during lunch hour. They're the real deal!

Prevention: Check out their Web site www.prevention.com. *Prevention* offers sound advice on many health and fitness topics.

Runner's World: This magazine always has great tips for runners and walkers and the latest news on gear. Visit www.runnersworld.com.

Shape: Find more information on this magazine at www.shape.com. *Shape* has recently changed editors and improved it's content. They're now offering terrific workout routines along with keeping up with the latest trends in the fitness world.

Yoga Journal: Visit www.yogajournal.com. This magazines offers information on types of yoga practices, yoga poses, as well as meditation, relaxation, retreats and yoga in your area.